Slow Cooker Poultry Recipes for Beginners

Delicious Meals for Carnivores

Roxana S. Hamilton

Sommario

INTRODUCTION

Hey there! Welcome to my book of dishes for the Crockery Pot.

My recipes are simply also scrumptious to maintain to myself. As well as it's the only cookbook you'll require to make one of the most scrumptious Crockery Pot recipes you've ever before tasted!

If there's one kitchen area home appliance I can not live without, it's my Crockery Pot. This gizmo has transformed my life entirely in the kitchen area! Gone are the days when I spent hrs every week, prepping and then cooking meals. And so lot of times those meals were unappetizing, with leftovers that nobody wished to eat.

Then along came my Crockery Pot Pressure Cooker ... and also currently I make delectable dishes everyday.

One of the biggest attractive functions of the Crock Pot is that it makes fresh and quick pleasant dishes in no time at all. Whether you're vegetarian or love your meat and hen, my publication has the most effective dishes for making fantastic, healthier meals. And ensure you make a luxurious rip off recipe on those days when you're not counting calories as well as fat! Those are the most effective dishes of all. In this book, I share my preferred.

Delicious BBQ Pulled Turkey

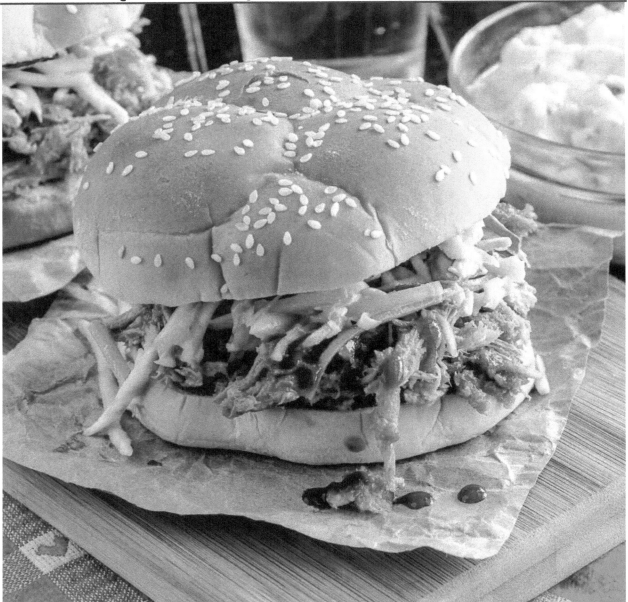

Ready in about: 100 minutes | Serves: 6 | Per serving: Calories 456; Carbs 19g; Fat 26g; Protein 37g

INGREDIENTS
2 pounds Turkey Breasts, boneless and skinless
1 cup Beer
1 ½ tbsp Oil
SAUCE:
2 tbsp Honey
½ cup Apple Cider Vinegar

1 tsp Liquid Smoke
2 tsp Sriracha
1 tsp Garlic Powder
1 tsp Onion Powder
½ cup Mustard
1 tbsp Worcestershire Sauce
2 tbsp Honey
1 tsp Mustard Powder
2 tbsp Olive Oil
DIRECTIONS

Heat the oil on SAUTÉ mode at High. Add turkey and brown on all sides.
Whisk together all the sauce ingredients in a small bowl. Add beef and sauce to the Pressure cooker. Stir to combine.

Seal the lid and cook for 45 minutes on MEAT/STEW mode at High. When ready, release the pressure quickly. Remove the turkey to a plate and shred with two forks.

Set to SAUTÉ, and cook until the sauce is reduced and thickened, lid off. Return the turkey and stir to coat well.

Balsamic Chicken Thighs with Pears

Ready in about: 30 minutes | Serves: 6 | Per serving: Calories 488; Carbs 11g; Fat 34g; Protein 33g

INGREDIENTS

6 large Chicken Thighs
½ cup Sweet Onions, chopped
3 small Pears, peeled and sliced
2 tbsp Balsamic Vinegar
3 tsp Butter
1 cup Chicken Broth
1 tsp Cayenne Pepper
Salt and Pepper, to taste

DIRECTIONS

Melt the butter on SAUTÉ mode at High. Add chicken and sprinkle with the spices. Brown on all sides. Stir in the remaining ingredients. Seal the lid and cook for 20 minutes on POULTRY at High.

When ready, release the pressure naturally, for 10 minutes, and serve immediately.

Cheesy Drumsticks in Marinara Sauce

Ready in about: 35 minutes | Serves: 4 | Per serving: Calories 588; Carbs 15g; Fat 43g; Protein 36g

INGREDIENTS

4 Chicken Drumsticks
1 cup Sour Cream
1 ¾ cups Marinara Sauce
1 cup grated Cheddar Cheese
½ Butter Stick
1 tsp Chipotle Powder
½ tsp Rosemary
Salt and Pepper, to taste

DIRECTIONS

Melt the butter on SAUTÉ at High. Add marinara, chipotle, rosemary, and chicken. Season with salt and pepper.

Seal the lid and cook for 20 minutes on POULTRY at High pressure. When ready, release the pressure naturally, for 10 minutes. Stir in the cheese and sour cream, and serve.

Turkey Thighs with Fig Sauce

Ready in about: 35 minutes | Serves: 6 | Per serving: Calories 455; Carbs 62g; Fat 8g; Protein 34g

INGREDIENTS

2 pounds Turkey Thighs, skinless
1 cup Carrots, sliced
1 Onion, chopped
4 Potatoes, cubed
¼ cup Balsamic Vinegar
12 dried Figs, halved
2 cups Chicken Broth
½ Celery Stalk, diced
Salt and Black Pepper, to taste

DIRECTIONS

Place carrots, onion, potatoes, celery and turkey inside the pressure cooker. Whisk together the remaining ingredients, except the figs, in a bowl and pour the mixture over the turkey.

Season with salt and pepper, and stir in the figs, and 1 cup of water. Seal the lid, and cook for 15 minutes on MEAT/STEW, at High. When done, do a natural release, for 10 minutes.

Remove the figs, turkey, and veggies to serving plates. To serve, strain the sauce that's left in the cooker, and pour over the turkey and veggies.

Creamy Chicken with Mushrooms and Carrots

Ready in about: 30 minutes | Serves: 6 | Per serving: Calories 603; Carbs 14g; Fat 31g; Protein 59g

INGREDIENTS

6 Chicken Breasts, boneless and skinless
1 Sweet Onion, diced
1 cup Water
8 ounces Mushrooms, sliced
1 can Cream of Mushroom Soup
1 pound Baby Carrots
1 tbsp Butter
1 tbsp Olive Oil
2 tbsp Heavy Cream

DIRECTIONS

Heat oil and butter on SAUTÉ mode at High, until melted. Add onions and mushrooms, and cook for 3 minutes, until soft. Stir in the carrots, add chicken, and pour mushroom soup, and water.

Seal the lid and cook for 8 minutes on BEANS/CHILI mode at High. When ready, do a quick pressure release and remove the mushrooms, chicken, and carrots to a plate.

In the pressure cooker, stir in the heavy cream and cook the sauce until it thickens, on SAUTÉ, for a few minutes. Serve the chicken and veggies drizzled with the sauce.

Turkey with Tomatoes and Red Beans

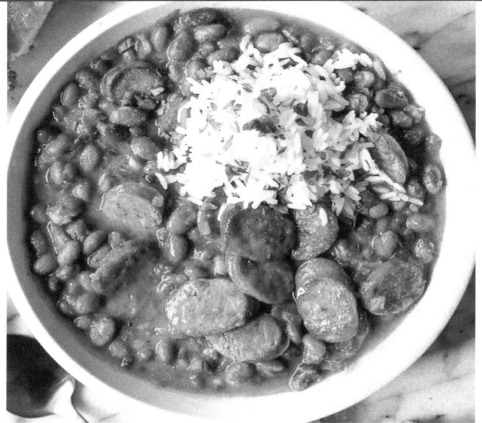

Ready in about: 20 minutes | Serves: 6 | Per serving: Calories 212; Carbs 12g; Fat 8g; Protein 23g

INGREDIENTS

1-pound Turkey Breast, cut into bite-sized cubes
1 (16 oz) can Stewed Tomatoes
1 (16 oz) can Red Kidney Beans, drained
2 cups Chicken Stock
½ cup Sour Cream
Salt and Black Pepper, to taste
2 tbsp Parsley, chopped

DIRECTIONS

Place beans, tomatoes, turkey, stock, and sour cream in your pressure cooker. Season to taste. Seal the lid, set on SOUP, cook for 20 minutes at High.

Release the pressure quickly. Sprinkle with freshly chopped parsley to serve.

Orange and Cranberry Turkey Wings

Ready in about: 40 minutes | Serves: 4 | Per serving: Calories 525; Carbs 20g; Fat 38g; Protein 26g

INGREDIENTS

1 pound Turkey Wings
¼ cup Orange Juice
1 stick Butter, softened
2 cups Cranberries
2 Onions, sliced
2 cups Vegetable Stock
½ tsp Cayenne Pepper
Salt and Pepper, to taste

DIRECTIONS

Melt the butter on SAUTÉ. Add the turkey wings, season with salt, pepper, and cayenne pepper, and cook until browned, for a few minutes. Stir in the remaining ingredients. Seal the lid.

Cook for 25 minutes on POULTRY at High. Release the pressure naturally, for 10 minutes, and serve.

Chicken Drumettes in Creamy Tomato Sauce

Ready in about: 25 minutes | Serves: 2 | Per serving: Calories 525; Carbs 21g; Fat 41g; Protein 28g

INGREDIENTS

2 Chicken Drumsticks, trimmed of fat
2 cups Tomato Sauce
1 cup Heavy Cream
1 cup sharp Parmesan cheese, grated
4 tbsp Butter
1 tsp Garlic paste
1 tsp Chipotle powder
1 tbsp fresh Basil leaves, chopped
Salt and ground Black Pepper, to taste
½ tsp fresh Rosemary, chopped

DIRECTIONS

Melt butter on SAUTÉ at High. Add garlic paste, chipotle, tomato sauce, rosemary, and basil. Sprinkle the chicken drumsticks with salt and ground black pepper. Place the chicken down into the sauce, so it resembles a nestle.

Seal the lid, select POULTRY and cook at High pressure for 20 minutes. Once it goes off, release the pressure naturally, for 10 minutes. Stir in the cheese and sour cream and serve right away.

Delicious Turkey Meatloaf

Ready in about: 30 minutes | Serves: 4 | Per serving: Calories 317; Carbs 7g; Fat 16g; Protein 37g

INGREDIENTS

1 ½ pounds ground Turkey
1 Carrot, grated
1 Onion, diced
1 Celery Stalk, diced
½ cup Breadcrumbs
1 Egg, cracked in the bowl
1 tsp Garlic, minced
½ tsp Thyme
¼ tsp Oregano
¼ tsp Salt
¼ tsp Black Pepper
1 tsp Worcestershire Sauce
1 ½ cups Water
Cooking spray, to grease

DIRECTIONS

Pour the water in your pressure cooker. Combine the remaining ingredients in a large bowl. Grease a baking pan with cooking spray and add in the mixture, pressing it tightly.

Lay the trivet and lower the pan on top of the trivet, inside your Pressure cooker. Seal the lid and cook on POULTRY de for 15 minutes at High. Do a natural release, for 10 minutes.

Spicy Rosemary Chicken

Ready in about: 55 minutes | Serves: 4 | Per serving: Calories 294; Carbs 4g; Fat 7g; Protein 50g

INGREDIENTS

1 Whole Chicken
1 tbsp Cayenne Pepper
2 Rosemary Sprigs
2 Garlic Cloves, crushed
¼ Onion, halved, or sliced
1 tsp dried Rosemary
Salt and Pepper, to taste
1 ½ cups Chicken Broth

DIRECTIONS

Wash and pat dry the chicken. Season with salt, pepper, rosemary, and cayenne pepper. Rub the spices onto the meat. Stir in onion, garlic, and rosemary sprig inside the chicken's cavity.

Place the chicken in the cooker, and pour in broth around the chicken, not over. Seal the lid and cook for 30 minutes on MEAT/STEW, at High. When done, let pressure drop naturally, for about 10 minutes.

Creamy Chicken in Beer Sauce

Ready in about: 40 minutes | Serves: 4 | Per serving: Calories 534; Carbs 9g; Fat 33g; Protein 46g

INGREDIENTS

1 ½ pounds Chicken Breasts
10 ounces Beer
1 cup Green Onions, chopped
1 ¼ cups Greek Yogurt
¼ cup Arrowroot
½ tsp Sage
2 tsp dried Thyme
2 tsp dried Rosemary
2 tbsp Olive Oil

DIRECTIONS

Heat the oil on SAUTÉ mode at High. Add onions and cook for 2 minutes. Coat the chicken with the arrowroot. Add the chicken to the cooker and cook until browned on all sides.

Pour the beer over and bring the mixture to a boil. Stir in the herbs and cook on SOUP for 30 minutes at High pressure. Do a quick release, and stir in yogurt before serving.

Barbecue Wings

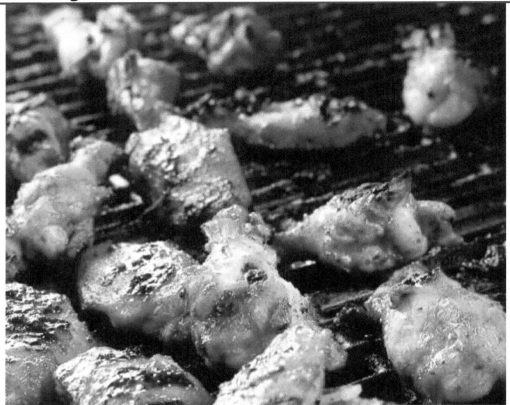

**Ready in about: 15 minutes | Serves: 4 | Per serving: Calories 140;
Carbs 2g; Fat 3g; Protein 19g**

INGREDIENTS
12 Chicken Wings
¼ cup Barbecue Sauce
1 cup of Water
DIRECTIONS
Place chicken wings and water in your pressure cooker. Seal the lid. Cook for 5 minutes on BEANS/CHILI at High. When ready, do a quick release.
Rinse under cold water and pat wings dry. Remove the liquid from the pot. Return the wings to the pressure cooker and pour in barbecue sauce. Mix with hands to coat them well.
Cook on SAUTÉ, lid off, on all sides, until sticky. Serve hot.

Lemon-Garlic Chicken Thights

Ready in about: 30 minutes | Serves: 4 | Per serving: Calories 487; Carbs 8g; Fat 36g; Protein 28g

INGREDIENTS

4 Chicken Thighs
1 ½ tbsp Olive Oil
½ tsp Garlic Powder
Salt and Black Pepper to taste
½ tsp Red Pepper Flakes
½ tsp Smoked Paprika
1 small Onion, chopped
2 cloves Garlic, sliced
½ cup Chicken Broth
1 tsp Italian Seasoning
1 Lemon, zested and juiced
1 ½ tbsp Heavy Cream
Lemon slices to garnish
Chopped parsley to garnish

DIRECTIONS

Warm the olive oil on SAUTÉ, and add the chicken thighs; cook to brown on each side for 3 minutes. Remove the browned chicken onto a plate. Add butter to the pot to melt, then, add garlic, onions, and lemon juice.

Stir them with a spoon to deglaze the bottom of the pot and let them cook for 1 minute. Add Italian seasoning, chicken broth, lemon zest, and the chicken. Seal the lid, select MEAT/STEW at High pressure for 15 minutes. Once the timer has ended, let the pot sit closed for 2 minutes, then do a quick pressure release. Open the lid.

Remove the chicken onto a plate and add the heavy cream to the pot. Select SAUTÉ and stir the cream into the sauce until it thickens.

Turn off the cooker and return the chicken. Coat the chicken with sauce. Dish the sauce into a serving platter and serve with the steamed kale and spinach mix. Garnish with the lemon and parsley.

Italian-Style Chicken Breasts with Kale Pesto

Ready in about: 30 minutes | Serves: 4 | Per serving: Calories 372; Carbs 5g; Fat 19g; Protein 35g

INGREDIENTS

4 Chicken Breasts, skinless and boneless
½ cup Heavy Cream
½ cup Chicken Broth
¼ tsp minced Garlic
Salt and Black Pepper to taste
¼ tsp Italian Seasoning
¼ cup Roasted Red Peppers
1 tbsp Tuscan Kale Pesto
1 tbsp Cornstarch

DIRECTIONS

Place the chicken at the bottom of the cooker. Pour the broth over, and add the Italian seasoning, garlic, salt, and pepper. Seal the lid, select MEAT/STEW mode at High pressure for 15 minutes.

Once the timer has ended, do a natural pressure release for 5 minutes, then a quick pressure release to let the remaining steam out, and open the pot.

Use a spoon to remove the chicken onto a plate and select SAUTÉ mode.

Scoop out any **fat** or unwanted chunks from the sauce. In a bowl, add cream, cornstarch, red peppers, and pesto.

Mix them with a spoon. Pour the creamy mixture into the pot and whisk it for 4 minutes until it is well mixed and thickened.

Put the chicken back in the pot and let it simmer for 3 minutes.

Turn the pot off and dish the sauce onto a serving platter. Serve the chicken with sauce over a bed of cooked quinoa.

Jasmine Rice and Chicken Taco Bowls

Ready in about: 20 minutes | Serves: 4 | Per serving: Calories 523; Carbs 41g; Fat 22g; Protein 44g

INGREDIENTS

4 Chicken Breasts
2 cups Chicken Broth
2 ¼ packets Taco Seasoning
1 cup Jasmine Rice
1 Green Bell Pepper, seeded and diced
1 Red Bell Pepper, seeded and diced
1 cup Salsa
Salt and Black Pepper to taste
To Serve:
Grated Cheese, of your choice
Chopped Cilantro
Sour Cream
Avocado Slices

DIRECTIONS

Pour in the chicken broth, add the chicken,and pour the taco seasoning over it. Add the salsa and stir it lightly with a spoon. Seal the lid and select MEAT/STEW at High setting for 15 minutes. Do a quick pressure release.
Add the rice and peppers, and use a spoon to push them into the sauce. Seal the lid, and select BEANS/CHILI mode on High pressure for 15 minutes.
Once the timer has ended, do a quick pressure release, and open the lid. Gently stir the mixture, adjust the taste with salt and pepper and spoon the chicken dish into serving bowls. Top it with some sour cream, avocado slices, sprinkle with chopped cilantro and some cheese, to serve.

Honey-Ginger Shredded Chicken

Ready in about: 35 minutes | Serves: 4 | Per serving: Calories 462; Carbs 38g; Fat 16g; Protein 37g

INGREDIENTS

4 Chicken Breasts, skinless
¼ cup Sriracha Sauce
2 tbsp Butter
1 tsp grated Ginger
2 cloves Garlic, minced
½ tsp Cayenne Pepper
½ tsp Red Chili Flakes
½ cup Honey
½ cup Chicken Broth
Salt and Black Pepper to taste
Chopped Scallion to garnish

DIRECTIONS

In a bowl, add chicken broth, honey, ginger, sriracha sauce, red pepper flakes, cayenne pepper, and garlic. Use a spoon to mix them well and set aside. Put the chicken on a plate and season them with salt and pepper. Set aside too. On the cooker, select SAUTÉ mode. Melt the butter, and add the chicken in 2 batches to brown on both sides for about 3 minutes. Add all the chicken back to the pot and pour the pepper sauce over it.

Seal the lid, select MEAT/STEW at High pressure for 20 minutes. Once the timer has ended, do a natural pressure release for 5 minutes, then a quick pressure release to let the remaining steam out, and open the lid.

Remove the chicken onto a cutting board and shred them using two forks. Plate the chicken in a serving bowl, pour the sauce over it, and garnish it with the scallions. Serve with a side of sauteéd mushrooms.

Coconut-Lime Chicken Curry

Ready in about: 35 minutes | Serves: 4 | Per serving: Calories 643; Carbs 30g; Fat 44g; Protein 42g

INGREDIENTS

4 Chicken Breasts
4 tbsp Red Curry Paste
½ cup Chicken Broth
2 cups Coconut Milk
4 tbsp Sugar
Salt and Black Pepper to taste
2 Red Bell Pepper, seeded and cut in 2-inch sliced
2 Yellow Bell Pepper, seeded and cut in 2-inch slices
2 cup Green Beans, cut in half
2 tbsp Lime Juice

DIRECTIONS

Add the chicken, red curry paste, salt, pepper, coconut milk, broth and swerve sugar. Seal the lid, select MEAT/STEW at High pressure for 15 minutes. Once the timer has ended, do a quick pressure release.

Remove the chicken onto a cutting board and select SAUTÉ. Add the bell peppers, green beans, and lime juice. Stir the sauce with a spoon and let it simmer for 4 minutes. Slice the chicken with a knife and return it to the pot. Stir and simmer for a minute. Dish the chicken with sauce and vegetable, and serve with coconut flatbread.

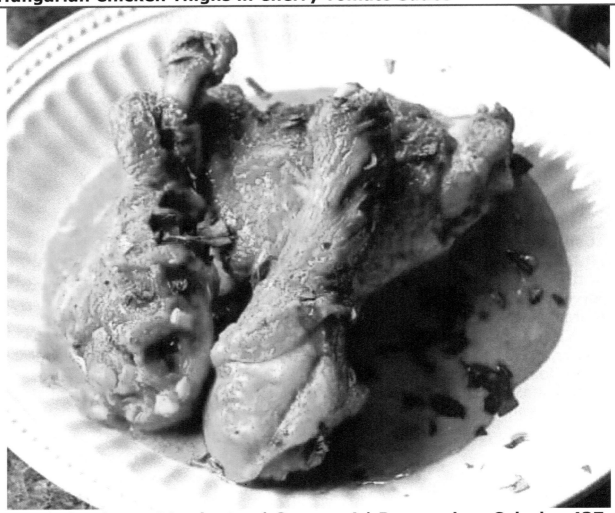

Ready in about: 30 minutes | Serves: 4 | Per serving: Calories 437; Carbs 8g; Fat 37g; Protein 24g

INGREDIENTS
4 Chicken Thighs, skinless but with bone
4 tbsp Olive Oil
1 cup Crushed Cherry Tomatoes
2 tbsp Hungarian Paprika
1 large Red Bell Pepper, seeded and diced
1 large Green Bell Pepper, seeded and diced
1 Red Onion, diced
Salt and Black Pepper to taste
1 tbsp chopped Basil
½ cup Chicken Broth
1 bay Leaf
½ tsp dried Oregano
DIRECTIONS

Place the chicken on a clean flat surface and season with hungarian paprika, salt and pepper. Select SAUTÉ mode, on the pressure cooker. Pour the oil in, once heated add the chicken. Brown on both sides for 6 minutes.

Then, add the onions and peppers. Cook until soft for 5 minutes. Add tomatoes, bay leaf, salt, broth, pepper, and oregano. Stir using a spoon.

Seal the lid, select MEAT/STEW mode at High pressure for 20 minutes.

Do a natural pressure release for 5 minutes, then a quick pressure release to let the remaining steam out.

Discard the bay leaf. Dish the chicken with the sauce into a serving bowl and garnish it with the chopped basil. Serve over a bed of steamed squash spaghetti.

Black Currant and Lemon Chicken

Ready in about: 20 minutes | Serves: 6 | Per serving: Calories 286; Carbs 8g; Fat 18g; Protein 25g

INGREDIENTS

1 ½ pound Chicken Breasts
¼ cup Red Currants
2 Garlic Cloves, minced
6 Lemon Slices
1 cup Scallions, chopped
1 cup Black Olives, pitted
2 tbsp Canola Oil
¼ tsp Pepper
1 tsp Coriander Seeds
1 tsp Cumin
¼ tsp Salt
2 ¼ cups Water

DIRECTIONS

Heat the oil on SAUTÉ at High. Add scallions, coriander, and garlic and cook for 30 seconds. Add the chicken and top with olives and red currants. Season with salt and pepper.

Arrange the lemon slices on top, and pour the water over. Seal the lid and cook on POULTRY for 15 minutes at High pressure. When ready, release the pressure naturally, for 10 minutes.

Buffalo Chicken Chili

Ready in about: 40 minutes | Serves: 4 | Per serving: Calories 487; Carbs 8g; Fat 34g; Protein 41g

INGREDIENTS

4 Chicken Breasts, boneless and skinless
½ cup Buffalo Sauce
2 large White Onion, finely chopped
2 cups finely chopped Celery
1 tbsp Olive Oil
1 tsp dried Thyme
3 cups Chicken Broth
1 tsp Garlic Powder
½ cup crumbled Blue Cheese + extra for serving
4 oz Cream Cheese, cubed in small pieces
Salt and Pepper, to taste

DIRECTIONS

Put the chicken on a clean flat surface and season with pepper and salt. Set aside. Select SAUTÉ mode. Heat olive oil, add the onion and celery. Sauté constantly stirring, until they soft and fragrant, for about 5 minutes.

Add the garlic powder and thyme. Stir and cook them for about a minute, and add the chicken, hot sauce, and chicken broth. Season with salt and pepper. Seal the lid, select MEAT/STEW at High pressure for 20 minutes. Meanwhile, add the blue cheese and cream cheese in a bowl, and use a fork to smash them together. Set the mixture aside. Once the timer has ended, do a natural pressure release for 5 minutes.

Remove chicken onto a flat surface with a slotted spoon and use forks to shred it; then return it back the pot. Select SAUTÉ mode. Add the cheese to the pot and stir until is slightly incorporated into the sauce.

Dish the buffalo chicken soup into bowls. Sprinkle the remaining cheese over and serve with sliced baguette.

Tuscany-Style Sund-Dried Tomato Chicken

Ready in about: 30 minutes | Serves: 4 | Per serving: Calories 576; Carbs 12g; Fat 44g; Protein 45g

INGREDIENTS

4 Chicken Thighs, cut into 1-inch pieces
1 tbsp Olive Oil
1 ½ cups Chicken Broth
Salt to taste
1 cup chopped Sun-Dried Tomatoes with Herbs
2 tbsp Italian Seasoning
2 cups Baby Spinach
¼ tsp Red Pepper Flakes
6 oz softened Cream Cheese, cut into small cubes
1 cup shredded Pecorino Cheese

DIRECTIONS

Pour the chicken broth in the cooker, and add Italian seasoning, chicken, tomatoes, salt, and red pepper flakes. Stir with a spoon. Seal the lid, select MEAT/STEW mode at High pressure for 15 minutes.

Once the timer has ended, do a quick pressure release, and open the lid. Add and stir in the spinach, parmesan cheese, and cream cheese until the cheese melts and is fully incorporated. Let it stay in the warm for 5 minutes. Dish the Tuscan chicken over a bed of zoodles or a side of steamed asparagus and serve.

Gorgeous Chicken Fajitas with Guacamole

Ready in about: 30 minutes | Serves: 4 | Per serving: Calories 423; Carbs 9g; Fat 22g; Protein 40g

INGREDIENTS

2 lb Chicken Breasts, skinless and cut in 1-inch slices
½ cup Chicken Broth
1 Yellow Onion, sliced
1 Green Bell Pepper, seeded and sliced
1 Yellow Bell Pepper, seeded and sliced
1 Red Bell Pepper, seeded and sliced
2 tbsp Cumin Powder
2 tbsp Chili Powder
Salt to taste
Half a Lime
Cooking Spray
Fresh cilantro, to garnish
<u>Assembling:</u>
Tacos, Guacamole, Sour Cream, Salsa, Cheese

DIRECTIONS

Grease the pot with cooking spray and line the bottom with the peppers and onion. Lay the chicken on the bed of peppers and sprinkle with salt, chili powder, and cumin powder. Squeeze some lime juice.

Pour the chicken broth over, seal the lid and select MEAT/STEW at High for 20 minutes. Once the timer has ended, do a quick pressure release. Dish the chicken with the vegetables and juice onto a large serving platter. Add the sour cream, cheese, guacamole, salsa, and tacos in one layer on the side of the chicken.

Mediterranean Chicken Meatballs

Ready in about: 30 minutes | Serves: 4 | Per serving: Calories 378; Carbs 13g; Fat 19g; Protein 26g

INGREDIENTS

1 lb Ground Chicken
1 Egg, cracked into a bowl
6 tsp Flour
Salt and Black Pepper to taste
2 tbsp chopped Basil + Extra to garnish
1 tbsp Olive Oil + ½ tbsp Olive Oil
1 ½ tsp Italian Seasoning
1 Red Bell Pepper, seeded and sliced
2 cups chopped Green Beans
½ lb chopped Asparagus
1 cup chopped Tomatoes
1 cup Chicken Broth

DIRECTIONS

In a mixing bowl, add chicken, egg, flour, salt, pepper, 2 tablespoons of basil, 1 tablespoon of olive oil, and Italian seasoning. Mix well with hands, and make 16 large balls out of the mixture. Set the meatballs aside.

Select SAUTÉ mode. Heat half teaspoon of olive oil, add the peppers, green beans, and asparagus. Cook for 3 minutes while stirring frequently. After 3 minutes, use a spoon the veggies onto a plate and set aside.

Heat the remaining oil, and then fry the meatballs in batches, for 2 minutes on each side to brown them lightly.Next, put all meatballs back to the pot along with the vegetables and chicken broth.

Seal the lid.

Select MEAT/STEW mode at High pressure for 15 minutes. Once it goes off, do a quick pressure release. Dish the meatballs with sauce into a serving bowl and garnish with basil. Serve with over cooked tagliatelle pasta.

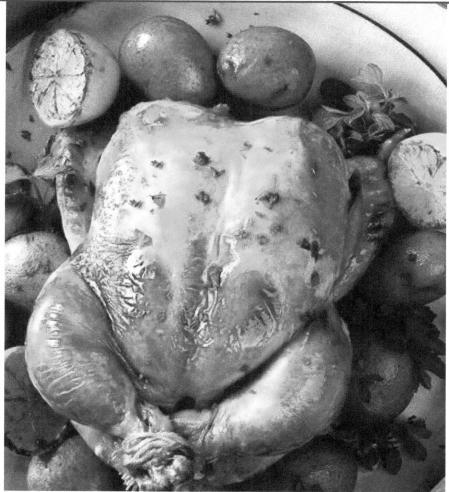

Ready in about: 60 minutes | Serves: 6 | Per serving: Calories 234; Carbs 5g; Fat 8g; Protein 33g

INGREDIENTS

1 medium Whole Chicken
1 Green Onion, minced
2 tbsp Sugar
1 tbsp Ginger, grated
2 tsp Soy Sauce
¼ cup White Wine
½ cup Chicken Broth
1 ½ tbsp Olive Oil
1 tsp Salt
¼ tsp Pepper

DIRECTIONS

Heat oil on SAUTÉ mode at High. Season the chicken with sugar and half the salt and pepper, and brown on all sides, for a few minutes. Remove from the cooker and set aside.

33

Whisk in together wine, broth, soy sauce, and salt. Add the chicken and seal the lid. Cook for 35 minutes on MEAT/STEW mode at High. When ready, release the pressure quickly.

Feta and Spinach Stuffed Chicken Breasts

Ready in about: 30 minutes | Serves: 4 | Per serving: Calories 417; Carbs 3g; Fat 27g; Protein 33g

INGREDIENTS

4 Chicken Breasts, skinless
Salt and Black Pepper to taste
1 cup Baby Spinach, frozen
½ cup crumbled Feta Cheese
½ tsp dried Oregano
½ tsp Garlic Powder
2 tbsp Olive Oil
2 tsp dried Parsley
1 cup Water

DIRECTIONS

Cover the chicken in plastic wrap and place on a cutting board.Use a rolling pin to pound flat to a quarter inch thickness. Remove the plastic wrap.

In a bowl, mix spinach, salt, feta cheese and scoop the mixture onto the chicken breasts. Wrap the chicken to secure the spinach filling in it. Use some toothpicks to secure the wrap firmly from opening.

Carefully season the chicken pieces with the oregano, parsley, garlic powder, and pepper. Set on SAUTÉ mode. Heat the oil, add the chicken to sear, until golden brown on each side. Work in 2 batches.

Remove the chicken onto a plate and set aside. Pour the water into the pot and use a spoon to scrape the bottom of the pot. Fit the steamer rack into the pot. Transfer the chicken onto the steamer rack.

Seal the lid and select MEAT/STEW at High pressure for 15 minutes. Once the timer has ended, do a quick pressure release. Plate the chicken and serve with a side of sautéed asparagus, and slices of tomatoes (optional).

Lemon-Garlic Chicken with Herby Stuffed

Ready in about: 50 minutes | Serves: 6 | Per serving: Calories 376; Carbs 5g; Fat 15g; Protein 48g

INGREDIENTS
4 lb Whole Chicken
1 tbsp Herbes de Provence Seasoning
1 tbsp Olive Oil
Salt and Black Pepper to season
2 cloves Garlic, peeled
1 tsp Garlic Powder
1 Yellow Onion, peeled and quartered
1 Lemon, quartered
1 ¼ cups Chicken Broth
DIRECTIONS
Put the chicken on a clean flat surface and pat it dry using paper towels. Sprinkle the top and cavity with salt, black pepper, and garlic powder. Stuff onion, lemon, Herbes de Provence, and garlic cloves into the cavity.
Arrange the steamer rack inside. Pour in the broth and place the chicken on the rack. Seal the lid, select MEAT/STEW at High for 30 minutes. Do a natural pressure release for 15 minutes, then a quick pressure release to let the remaining steam out. Remove the chicken onto a prepared baking pan, and to a preheat oven to 350 F.
Broil chicken for 5 minutes untol golden brown color on each side. Dish on a bed of steamed mixed veggies.

Fennel Chicken Breast

Ready in about: 25 minutes | Serves: 8 | Per serving: Calories 422; Carbs 3g; Fat 22g; Protein 51g

INGREDIENTS

2 pounds Chicken Breasts, boneless and skinless
1 cup Celery, chopped
1 cup Fennel, chopped
2 ¼ cups Chicken Stock
Salt and Pepper, to taste

DIRECTIONS

Chop the chicken into small pieces and place in your pressure cooker. Add the remaining ingredients and stir well to combine. Seal the lid, and set to BEANS/CHILI for 15 minutes at High.

When ready, release the pressure naturally, for 10 minutes. Season with salt and pepper, to taste.

BBQ Sticky Drumettes

Ready in about: 30 minutes | Serves: 4 | Per serving: Calories 374; Carbs 3g; Fat 11g; Protein 38g

INGREDIENTS

2 lb Chicken Drumettes, bone in and skin in
½ cup Chicken Broth
½ tsp Dry Mustard
½ tsp Sweet Paprika
½ tbsp. Cumin Powder
½ tsp Onion Powder
¼ tsp Cayenne Powder
Salt and Pepper, to taste
1 stick Butter, sliced in 5 to 7 pieces
BBQ Sauce to taste
Cooking Spray

DIRECTIONS

Pour the chicken broth in and insert the trivet. In a zipper bag, pour in dry mustard, cumin powder, onion powder, cayenne powder, salt, and pepper. Add the chicken, then zip, close the bag and shake it to coat the chicken well with the spices. You can toss the chicken in the spices in batches too.

After, remove the chicken from the bag and place on the steamer rack. Top with butter slices, seal the lid, select MEAT/STEW mode at High pressure for 20 minutes. Meanwhile, preheat an oven to 350 F.

Once it goes off, do a quick pressure release, and open the lid. Remove the chicken onto a clean flat cutting board and brush with barbecue sauce.

Grease a baking tray with cooking spray and arrange the chicken pieces on it.

Tuck the tray into the oven and broil the chicken for 4 minutes while paying close attention to prevent burning.

Herby Balsamic Chicken

Ready in about: 50 minutes | Serves: 4 | Per serving: Calories 412; Carbs 13g; Fat 16g; Protein 38g

INGREDIENTS

2 lb Chicken Thighs, bone in and skin on
2 tbsp Olive Oil
Salt and Pepper, to taste
1 ½ cups diced Tomatoes
¾ cup Yellow Onion
2 tsp minced Garlic
½ cup Balsamic Vinegar
3 tsp chopped fresh Thyme
1 cup Chicken Broth
2 tbsp chopped Oregano

DIRECTIONS

Using paper towels, pat dry the chicken and season with salt and pepper. Select SAUTÉ mode. Warm the olive and add the chicken with skin side down. Cook to golden brown on each side, for about 9 minutes. Set aside. Then, add the onions and tomatoes, and sauté them for 3 minutes while stirring occasionally. Top the onions with the garlic, and cook for 30 seconds, until fragrant Stir in chicken broth, salt, thyme, and balsamic vinegar.

Add back the chicken, seal the lid, and set on MEAT/STEW at High pressure for 20 minutes. Meanwhile, preheat oven to 350 F. Do a quick pressure release. Remove the chicken to a baking tray and leave the sauce inside the pot to thicken for about 10 minutes, on SAUTÉ mode. Tuck the baking tray in the oven and let the chicken broil on each side until golden brown, for about 5 minutes. Remove and set aside to cool slightly.

Adjust the seasoning of the sauce and cook the sauce until desired thickness. Place chicken in a serving bowl and drizzle the sauce all over. Garnish with parsley and serve with roasted tomatoes, carrots, and sweet potatoes.

Effortless Coq Au Vin

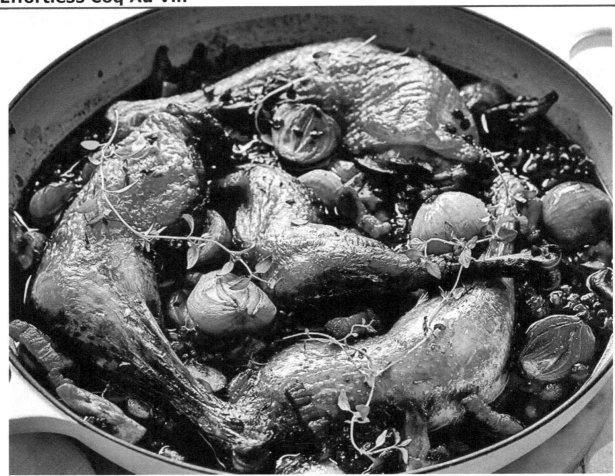

Ready in about: 60 minutes | Serves: 8 | Per serving: Calories 538; Carbs 40g; Fat 30g; Protein 26g

INGREDIENTS

2 pounds Chicken Thighs
4 ounces Bacon, chopped
14 ounces Red Wine
1 cup Parsley, chopped
2 Onions, chopped
4 small Potatoes, halved
7 ounces White Mushrooms, sliced
1 tsp Garlic Paste
2 tbsp Flour
¼ cup Olive Oil
2 tbsp Cognac
Salt and Black Pepper, to taste
Water, as needed

DIRECTIONS

Heat oil on SAUTÉ mode at High, and brown the chicken on all sides. Then, set aside. Add in onion, garlic, and bacon and cook for 2 minutes, until soft. Whisk in the flour and cognac.
Stir in the remaining ingredients, except for the mushrooms. Add enough water to cover everything. Seal the lid, press SOUP mode and cook for 20 minutes at High. When cooking is over, release the pressure quickly.
Stir in the mushrooms, seal the lid and cook for 5 more minutes on STEAM at High. Do a quick pressure release

Cajun Chicken and Green Beans

INGREDIENTS

4 boneless and skinless Chicken Breasts, frozen

2 cups Green Beans, frozen

14 ounces Cornbread Stuffing

1 tsp Cajun Seasoning

1 cup Chicken Broth

DIRECTIONS

Combine the chicken and broth in the cooker, seal the lid, and cook on POULTRY for 20 minutes at High. Do a quick pressure release. Add the green beans, seal the lid again, and cook for 2 more minutes on STEAM at High. Do a quick release, stir in the cornbread stuffing and Cajun seasoning and cook for another 5 minutes, on SAUTÉ, lid off. When ready, release the pressure quickly.

Turkey Breasts in Maple and Habanero Sauce

Ready in about: 30 minutes | Serves: 4 | Per serving: Calories 446; Carbs 23g; Fat 16g; Protein 51g

INGREDIENTS

2 pounds Turkey Breasts
6 tbsp Habanero Sauce
½ cup Tomato Puree
¼ cup Maple Syrup
1 ½ cups Water
½ tsp Cumin
1 tsp Smoked Paprika
Salt and Black Pepper, to taste

DIRECTIONS

Pour the water in your pressure cooker and place the turkey inside. Season with salt and black pepper. Seal the lid, press POULTRY for 15 minutes at High pressure. Release the pressure naturally, for 10 minutes.

Discard cooking liquid. Shred turkey inside the cooker and add the remaining ingredients. Cook on SAUTÉ at High, lid off, for a few minutes, until thickened.

Greek-Style Chicken Legs with Herbs

Ready in about: 35 minutes | Serves: 4 | Per serving: Calories 317; Carbs 15g; Fat 16g; Protein 28g

INGREDIENTS

4 Chicken Legs, skinless
1 cup Onions, thinly sliced
2 ripe Tomatoes, chopped
1 tsp Garlic, minced
2 tbsp corn Flour
1 ½ cups Chicken broth
3 tsp Olive Oil
1 tsp ground Cumin
2 tsp dried Rosemary
Salt and ground Black Pepper
½ cup Feta Cheese, cubes for garnish
10 Black Olives for garnish

DIRECTIONS

Season the chicken with salt, black pepper, rosemary, and cumin. Heat oil on SAUTÉ mode at High. Brown the chicken legs, for 3 minutes per side. Stir in the onions and cook for another 4 minutes.

Add the garlic and cook for another minute. In a measuring cup, stir the corn flour into the stock to make a slurry. When mixed, add the stock to the chicken. Add the tomatoes and give it a good stir.

Seal the lid and switch the pressure release valve to close. Hit POULTRY and set to 20 minutes at High. Once it goes off, release the pressure quickly. Serve with a side of feta cheese and black olives.

Chicken Stew with Shallots and Carrots

Ready in about: 25 minutes | Serves: 6 | Per serving: Calories 305; Carbs 15g; Fat 5g; Protein 39g

INGREDIENTS

1 cup Chicken Stock 3 tsp Vegetable Oil
3 Carrots, peeled, cored, and sliced
6 Shallots, halved and thinly sliced
½ tsp ground Black Pepper
1 tsp Cayenne Pepper
1 tsp Salt
10 boneless, skinless Chicken Thighs, trimmed bone-in, skin-on
2 tbsp Balsamic Vinegar
1 tbsp chopped fresh Parsley, for garnish

DIRECTIONS

Sprinkle the chicken with the salt, cayenne pepper, and black pepper. Select SAUTÉ at High and heat the oil. Add in the thighs and brown lightly on both sides, turning once or twice. Set it aside.

Add the remaining ingredients. Dip the browned chicken in the mixture. Seal the lid and cook for 20 minutes on POULTRY at Hgh Pressure. Allow for a natural pressure release, for 10 minutes, sprinkle with parsley and serve.

Thyme and Lemon Drumsticks with Red Sauce

Ready in about: 35 minutes | Serves: 4 | Per serving: Calories 268; Carbs 2g; Fat 16g; Protein 26g

INGREDIENTS

4 Chicken Drumsticks, fresh
1 Onion, sliced
½ cup canned, diced, Tomatoes
2 tsp dried Thyme
1 tsp Lemon Zest
½ cup Water
2 tbsp Lemon Juice
1 tbsp Olive Oil
Salt and Black Pepper, to taste

DIRECTIONS

Heat oil on SAUTÉ at High. Add drumsticks and cook them for a few minutes, until lightly browned. Stir in the remaining ingredients. Seal the lid and cook for 15 minutes on POULTRY at High.

Once cooking is complete, release the pressure naturally, for 10 minutes. Serve immediately.

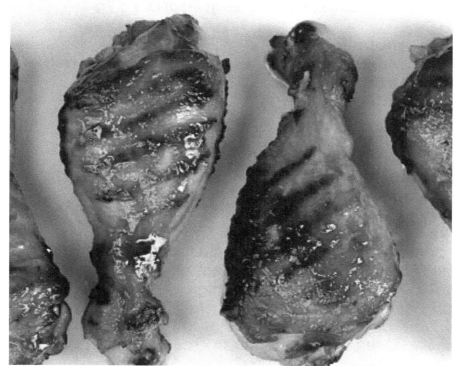

Ready in about: 30 minutes | Serves: 4 | Per serving: Calories 418; Carbs 7g; Fat 18g; Protein 53g

INGREDIENTS

4 Chicken Legs about 8-ounce each
1 Onion, chopped
1 Tomato, chopped
½ cup Sour Cream
1 cup Chicken Broth
1 tbsp Olive Oil
2 tsp Smoked Paprika
½ tsp Garlic Powder
¼ tsp Salt
¼ tsp Black Pepper

DIRECTIONS

Season the chicken with salt, black pepper, garlic powder, and smoked paprika, in a big bowl. Heat the oil on SAUTÉ at High, and add the seasoned chicken legs.

Cook until browned on all sides. Stir in the remaining ingredients and seal the lid. Cook for 15 minutes on MEAT/STEW at High. When ready, release the pressure naturally, for 15 minutes.

Creamy and Garlicky Chicken

Ready in about: 25 minutes | Serves: 4 | Per serving: Calories 455; Carbs 3g; Fat 26g; Protein 57g

INGREDIENTS

1 cup Spinach, chopped
2 lbs Chicken Breasts, boneless and skinless, cut in half
¾ cup Chicken Broth
2 Garlic Cloves, minced
2 tbsp Olive Oil
¾ cup Heavy Cream
½ cup Sun-Dried Tomatoes
2 tsp Italian Seasoning
½ cup Parmesan Chicken
½ tsp Salt

DIRECTIONS

In a small bowl, combine oil with garlic, salt, and seasonings. Rub the chicken on all sides with this mixture. Heat oil and brown the chicken on all sides, about 4-5 minutes, on SAUTÉ at High.

Pour the broth in and seal the lid. Press MEAT/STEW and cook for 20 minutes at High pressure. After 9 minutes, hit CANCEL and do a quick pressure release. Open the lid and stir in cream.

Let simmer for 5 minutes with the lid off, on SAUTÉ at High, and then stir in the cheese. Add in tomatoes and spinach and cook just until the spinach wilts. Serve and enjoy.

Asian-style Sweet Chicken Drumsticks

Ready in about: 25 minutes | Serves: 4 | Per serving: Calories 384; Carbs 26g; Fat 19g; Protein 25g

INGREDIENTS

4 Chicken Drumsticks
1 cup Pineapples, chopped
½ cup Coconut Milk
½ cup Tomato Sauce
2 tbsp Brown Sugar
2 tbsp Apple Cider Vinegar
1 tbsp Lime Juice
4 tbsp Water
Salt and Pepper, to taste

DIRECTIONS

In a bowl, whisk together all ingredients, except for the chicken and pineapples. Place the chicken drumsticks and pineapples in the pressure cooker and pour the sauce over.

Seal the lid, set to MEAT/STEW, and adjust the cooking time to 15 minutes at High. Once the cooking is complete, do a quick pressure release. Give it a good stir before serving hot!

Mexican Cheesy Turkey Breasts

Ready in about: 25 minutes | Serves: 4 | Per serving: Calories 404; Carbs 20g; Fat 12g; Protein 50g

INGREDIENTS

24 ounces Turkey Breasts, frozen
1 cup shredded Mozzarella Cheese
1 cup mild Salsa
½ cup Chicken Broth
1 cup Tomato Sauce
3 tbsp Lime Juice
Salt and Pepper, to taste

DIRECTIONS

Place the tomato sauce, salsa, broth, lime juice, and turkey in your pressure cooker. Seal the lid, and cook on MEAT/STEW for 15 minutes at High.

Do a natural pressure release, for 10 minutes. Shred the turkey inside the cooker, and stir in the cheese. Cook for 1 minute on SAUTÉ, to melt cheese.

Sweet Potato & Chicken Curry

Ready in about: 30 minutes | Serves: 4 | Per serving: Calories 343; Carbs 19g; Fat 15g; Protein 26g

INGREDIENTS

1 pound Boneless and Skinless Chicken Breast, cubed
2 cups cubed Sweet Potatoes
2 cups Green Beans
½ Onion, chopped
1 Bell Pepper, sliced
1 ½ tsp Garlic, minced
1 tsp Cumin
1 cup Milk
2 tsp Butter
3 tbsp Curry Powder
1 tsp Turmeric
½ cup Chicken Broth
Salt and Pepper, to taste

DIRECTIONS

Melt butter on SAUTÉ mode at High. Add the onions and cook for about 3 minutes, until soft. Add the garlic and cook for 30 seconds more. Add the remaining ingredients, except the milk.

Stir well to combine and seal the lid. Hit BEANS/CHILI, and set to 12 minutes at High. Do a quick pressure release. Stir in the milk and set to SAUTÉ at High. Cook for 3 minutes, lid off. Serve immediately.

Chicken with Water Chestnuts

Ready in about: 15 minutes | Serves: 4 | Per serving: Calories 274; Carbs 11g; Fat 8g; Protein 32g

INGREDIENTS

1 pound Ground Chicken
¼ cup Chicken Broth
2 tbsp Balsamic Vinegar
½ cup Water Chestnuts, sliced
¼ cup Soy Sauce
A pinch of Allspice

DIRECTIONS

Place all ingredients in your pressure cooker. Give the mixture a good stir to combine. Seal the lid, and hit BEANS/CHILI mode.

Set the cooking time to 10 minutes at High pressure. Quick-release the pressure.

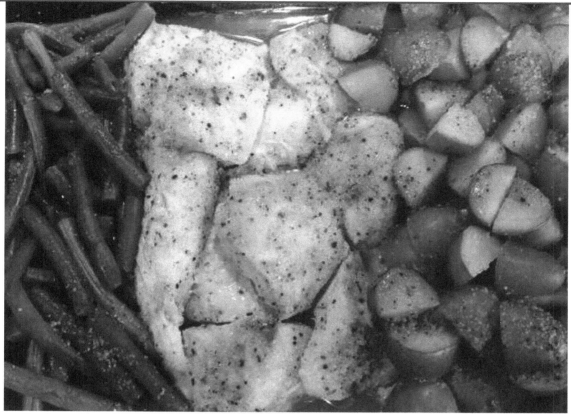

Ready in about: 30 minutes | Serves: 6 | Per serving: Calories 467; Carbs 16g; Fat 33g; Protein 32g

INGREDIENTS
2 pounds Chicken Thighs
1 tbsp Butter
¼ tsp dried Parsley
¼ tsp dried Oregano
½ tsp dried Thyme
Juice of 1 Lemon
½ cup Chicken Broth
2 tbsp Olive Oil
1 Garlic Clove, minced
1 pound Green Beans
1 pound Red Potatoes, halved
DIRECTIONS
Heat oil and butter on SAUTÉ at High, and cook until they melt. Add the minced garlic and cook for a minute. Place the chicken thighs inside and cook them on both sides, until golden.

Stir in the herbs and the lemon juice and cook for an additional minute, until fragrant. Add all remaining ingredients and stir well to combine. Seal the lid, and cook on BEANS/CHILI at High for 15 minutes.

After you hear the beep, release the pressure quickly. Serve immediately.

Creamy Southern Chicken

Ready in about: 25 minutes | Serves: 4 | Per serving: Calories 291; Carbs 32g; Fat 8g; Protein 31g

INGREDIENTS

1 ½ pounds Boneless Chicken Thighs
2 tsp Paprika
2 Bell Peppers, sliced
1 cup Chicken Broth
½ cup Milk
1 tbsp Chili Powder
¼ cup Lime Juice
1 tsp Cumin
½ tsp Garlic Powder
½ tsp Onion Powder
1 tsp Ground Coriander
½ tsp Cayenne Pepper
1 tbsp Olive Oil
1 tbsp Cornstarch

DIRECTIONS

Warm oil, and cook until hot and sizzling. Meanwhile, combine all spices in a small bowl and rub the mixture all over the chicken. Add the chicken, and cook until golden on both sides.

Pour broth and lime juice over, and stir in the peppers. Seal the lid, set the timer to 7 minutes on BEANS/CHILI at High. Do a quick release. Stir in milk and cornstarch and press SAUTÉ at High. Cook until the sauce thickens.

Easy Chicken Soup

Ready in about: 30 minutes | Serves: 6 | Per serving: Calories 272; Carbs 9g; Fat 11g; Protein 33g

INGREDIENTS

1 ½ pounds Boneless and Skinless Chicken Breasts
1 tbsp Chili Powder
2 tsp Garlic, minced
2 cups Chicken Broth
½ cup Water
1 tbsp Cumin
½ tsp Smoked Paprika
1 tsp Oregano
14 ounces canned diced Tomatoes
1 Bell Pepper, sliced
1 Onion, sliced

DIRECTIONS

Place all ingredients in your pressure cooker. Stir well to combine everything and seal the lid. Select BEANS/CHILI, set the timer to 20 minutes, at High. Do a natural pressure release, for about 10 minutes.

Pear and Onion Goose

Ready in about: 35 minutes | Serves: 6 | Per serving: Calories 313; Carbs 14g; Fat 8g; Protein 38g

INGREDIENTS

2 cups Chicken Broth
1 tbsp Butter
½ cup slice Onions
1 ½ pounds Goose, chopped into large pieces
2 tbsp Balsamic Vinegar
1 tsp Cayenne Pepper
3 Pears, peeled and sliced
¼ tsp Garlic Powder
½ tsp Pepper

DIRECTIONS

Melt the butter on SAUTÉ. Add the goose and cook until it becomes golden on all sides. Transfer to a plate. Add the onions and cook for 2 minutes. Return the goose to the cooker.

Add the rest of the ingredients, stir well to combine and seal the lid. Select BEANS/CHILI mode, and set the timer to 18 minutes at High pressure. Do a quick pressure release. Serve and enjoy!

Chicken Piccata

Ready in about: 20 minutes | Serves: 6 | Per serving: Calories 318; Carbs 15g; Fat 19g; Protein 19g

INGREDIENTS

6 Chicken Breast Halves
¼ cup Olive Oil
¼ cup Freshly Squeezed Lemon Juice
1 tbsp Sherry Wine
½ cup Flour
4 Shallots, chopped
3 Garlic Cloves, crushed
¾ cup Chicken Broth
1 tsp dried Basil
2 tsp Salt
¼ cup grated Parmesan Cheese
1 tbsp Flour
¼ cup Sour Cream
1 cup Pimento Olives, minced
¼ tsp White Pepper

DIRECTIONS

In a small bowl combine flour with some salt and pepper. Dip the chicken into flour and shake off the excess. Warm olive oil and brown the chicken on all sides for 3-4 minutes, on SAUTÉ at High.

Remove to a plate and set aside. Add shallots, and garlic and sauté for 2 minutes. Stir in sherry, broth, lemon juice, salt, olives, basil, and pepper. Return the chicken and any juices to the cooker.

Seal the lid, set to POULTRY and cook for 20 minutes at High. Do a quick pressure release. Stir in sour cream and parmesan.

Stewed Chicken with Kale

Ready in about: 30 minutes | Serves: 6 | Per serving: Calories 280; Carbs 14g; Fat 15g; Protein 21g

INGREDIENTS

1 pound Ground Chicken
1 cup Tomatoes, chopped
1 cup diced Onions
1 cup Carrots, chopped
1 cup Kale, chopped
½ cup Celery, chopped
6 cups Chicken Broth
2 Thyme Sprigs
1 tbsp Olive Oil
1 tsp Red Pepper Flakes
10 ounces Potato Noodles

DIRECTIONS

Warm oil on SAUTÉ mode at High. Add the chicken and cook until golden. Stir in the onions, carrots, and celery, and cook for about 5 minutes. Stir in the remaining ingredients, except the noodles.

Seal the lid, press BEANS/CHILI, and cook for 6 minutes at High. Do a quick pressure release. Stir in the potato noodles and seal the lid again. Cook at High pressure for 4 minutes. Do a quick pressure release, and serve hot.

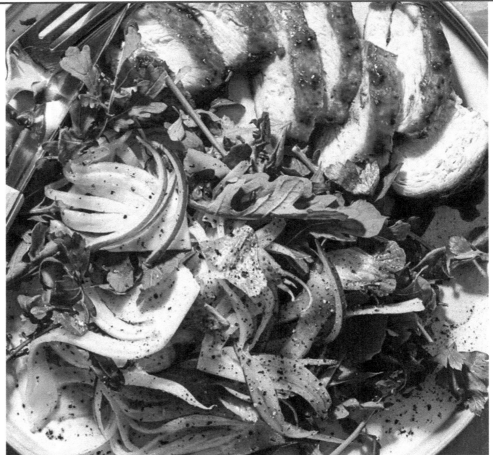

Ready in about: 25 minutes | Serves: 6 | Per serving: Calories 272; Carbs 7g; Fat 4g; Protein 48g

INGREDIENTS

2 pounds Boneless and Skinless Turkey Breast
1 cup Fennel Bulb, chopped
1 cup Celery with leaves, chopped
2 ¼ cups Chicken Stock
¼ tsp Pepper
¼ tsp Garlic Powder

DIRECTIONS

Throw all ingredients in your pressure cooker. Give it a good stir and seal the lid. Press BEANS/CHILI, and cook for 15 minutes at High. Do a quick pressure release. Shred the turkey with two forks.

Mexican Chicken

INGREDIENTS

1 Red Bell Pepper, diced
1 Green Bell Pepper, diced
1 Jalapeno, diced
2 pounds Chicken Breasts
10 ounces canned diced Tomatoes, undrained
1 Red Onion, diced
½ tsp Cumin
¾ tsp Chili Powder
¼ tsp Pepper
Juice of 1 Lime
½ cup Chicken Broth
1 tbsp Olive Oil

DIRECTIONS

Heat oil on SAUTÉ mode at High. When sizzling, add the onion and bell peppers and cook for about 3-4 minutes, until soft.

Add the remaining ingredients and give it a good stir to combine. Seal the lid, press POULTRY set for 15 minutes at High. After it beeps, release the pressure quickly.

Shred the chicken inside the pot with two forks, then stir to combine it with the juices. Serve and enjoy!

Chicken in Roasted Red Pepper Sauce

Ready in about: 25 minutes | Serves: 6 | Per serving: Calories 207; Carbs 5g; Fat 7g; Protein 32g

INGREDIENTS

1 ½ pounds Chicken Breasts, cubed
1 Onion, diced
4 Garlic Cloves
12 ounces Roasted Red Peppers
2 tsp Adobo Sauce
½ cup Beef Broth
1 tbsp Apple Cider Vinegar
1 tsp Cumin
Juice of ½ Lemon
3 tbsp chopped Cilantro
1 tbsp Olive Oil
Salt and Pepper, to taste

DIRECTIONS

Place garlic, red pepper, adobo sauce, lemon juice, vinegar, cilantro, and some salt and pepper, in a food processor. Process until the mixture becomes smooth. Set your pressure cooker to SAUTÉ at High and heat the oil.

Add the onion and cook for 2 minutes. Add the chicken cubes and cook until they are no longer pink. Pour sauce and broth over. Seal the lid, press BEANS/CHILI button, and set the timer to 8 minutes at High pressure. After you hear the beeping sound, do a quick pressure release. Serve and enjoy!

Turkey and Potatoes with Buffalo Sauce

Ready in about: 30 minutes | Serves: 4 | Per serving: Calories 377; Carbs 32g; Fat 9g; Protein 14g

INGREDIENTS
3 tbsp Olive Oil
4 tbsp Buffalo Sauce
1 pound Sweet Potatoes, cut into cubes
1 ½ pounds Turkey Breast, cut into pieces
½ tsp Garlic Powder
1 Onion, diced
½ cup Water

DIRECTIONS
Heat 1 tbsp of olive oil on SAUTÉ mode at High. Stir-fry onion in hot oil for about 3 minutes. Stir in the remaining ingredients.

Seal the lid, set to MEAT/STEW mode for 20 minutes at High pressure. When cooking is over, do a quick pressure release, by turning the valve to "open" position.

Fall-Off-Bone Chicken Drumsticks

Ready in about: 45 minutes | Serves: 3 | Per serving: Calories 454; Carbs 7g; Fat 27g; Protein 43g

INGREDIENTS
1 tbsp Olive Oil
6 Skinless Chicken Drumsticks
4 Garlic Cloves, smashed
½ Red Bell Pepper, diced
½ Onion, diced
2 tbsp Tomato Paste
2 cups Water

DIRECTIONS
Warm olive oil, and sauté onion and bell pepper, for about 4 minutes, on SAUTÉ at High. Add garlic and cook until golden, for a minute.
Combine the paste with water and pour into the cooker. Arrange the drumsticks inside. Seal the lid, set to POULTRY mode for 20 minutes at High pressure. When it beeps, do a quick pressure release. Serve immediately.

Coconut Chicken with Tomatoes

Ready in about: 25 minutes | Serves: 4 | Per serving: Calories 278; Carbs 28g; Fat 8g; Protein 19g

INGREDIENTS

1 ½ pounds Chicken Thighs
1 ½ cups chopped Tomatoes
1 Onion, chopped
1 ½ tbsp Butter
2 cups Coconut Milk
½ cup chopped Almonds
2 tsp Paprika
1 tsp Garam Masala
2 tbsp Cilantro, chopped
1 tsp Turmeric
1 tsp Cayenne Powder
1 tsp Ginger Powder
1 ¼ tsp Garlic Powder
Salt and Pepper, to taste

DIRECTIONS

Melt butter on SAUTÉ at High. Add the onions and sauté until translucent, for about 3 minutes. Add all spices, and cook for an additional minute, until fragrant. Stir in the tomatoes and coconut milk.

Place the chicken thighs inside and seal the lid. Cook on BEANS/CHILI on High pressure for 13 minutes. When it goes off, do a quick pressure release. Serve topped with chopped almonds and cilantro.

Cherry Tomato and Basil Chicken Casserole

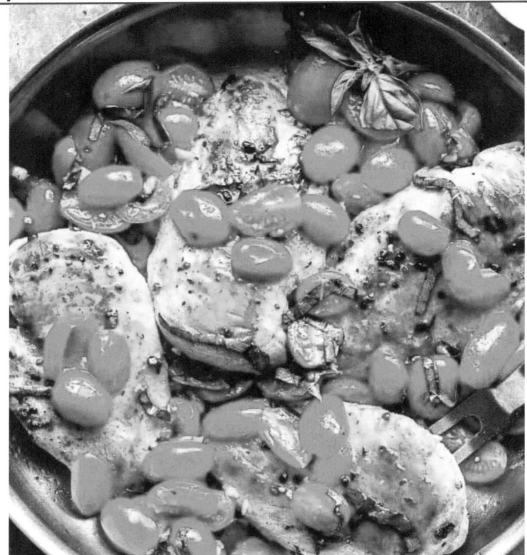

**Ready in about: 30 minutes | Serves: 4 | Per serving: Calories 337;
Carbs 12g; Fat 21g; Protein 27g**

INGREDIENTS
8 small Chicken Thighs
½ cup Green Olives
1 pound Cherry Tomatoes
1 cup Water
A handful of Fresh Basil Leaves
1 ½ tsp Garlic, minced
1 tsp dried Oregano
1 tbsp Olive Oil
DIRECTIONS

Season chicken with salt and pepper. Melt butter on SAUTÉ at High, and brown the chicken for about 2 minutes per side. Place tomatoes in a plastic bag and smash with a meat pounder.

Remove the chicken to a plate.

Combine tomatoes, garlic, water, and oregano in the pressure cooker. Top with the chicken and seal the lid. Cook on POULTRY at High for 15 minutes. When ready, do a quick pressure release. Stir in the basil and olives.

Sweet and Smoked Slow Cooked Turkey

Ready in about: 4 hours 15 minutes | Serves: 4 | Per serving:
Calories 513; Carbs 15 g; Fat 42g; Protein 65g

INGREDIENTS

1.5 pounds Turkey Breast
2 tsp Smoked Paprika
1 tsp Liquid Smoke
1 tbsp Mustard
3 tbsp Honey
2 Garlic Cloves, minced
4 tbsp Olive Oil
1 cup Chicken Broth

DIRECTIONS

Brush the turkey breast with olive oil and brown it on all sides, for 3-4 minutes, on SAUTÉ at High. Pour the chicken broth and all remaining ingredients in a bowl. Stir to combine.

Pour the mixture over the meat. Seal the lid, set on SLOW COOK mode for 4 hours. Do a quick pressure release.

Chicken and Beans Casserole with Chorizo

Ready in about: 35 minutes | Serves: 5 | Per serving: Calories 587; Carbs 52g; Fat 29g; Protein 29g

INGREDIENTS

1 tsp Garlic, minced
1 cup Onions, chopped
1 pound Chorizo Sausage, cut into pieces
4 Chicken Thighs, boneless, skinless
3 tbsp Olive Oil
2 cups Chicken Stock
11 ounces Asparagus, quartered
1 tsp Paprika
½ tsp ground Black Pepper
1 tsp Salt
2 Jalapeno Peppers, stemmed, cored, and chopped
26 oz canned whole Tomatoes, roughly chopped
1 ½ cups Kidney Beans

DIRECTIONS

On SAUTÉ, heat the oil and brown the sausage, for about 5 minutes per side. Transfer to a large bowl. In the same oil, add the thighs and brown them for 5 minutes. Remove to the same bowl as the sausage.

In the cooker, stir in onions and peppers. Cook for 3 minutes. Add in garlic and cook for 1 minute. Stir in the tomatoes, beans, stock, asparagus, paprika, salt, and black pepper.

Return the reserved sausage and thighs to the cooker. Stir well. Seal the lid and cook for 10 minutes on BEANS/CHILI mode at High Pressure. When ready, do a quick release and serve hot.

Creamy Turkey Breasts with Mushrooms

Ready in about: 35 minutes | Serves: 4 | Per serving: Calories 192; Carbs 5g; Fat 12g; Protein 15g

INGREDIENTS

20 ounces Turkey Breasts, boneless and skinless
6 ounces White Button Mushrooms, sliced
3 tbsp Shallots, chopped
½ tsp dried Thyme
¼ cup dry White Wine
cup Chicken Stock
1 Garlic Clove, minced
2 tbsp Olive Oil
3 tbsp Heavy Cream
1 ½ tbsp Cornstarch
Salt and Pepper, to taste

DIRECTIONS

Warm half of the olive oil on SAUTÉ mode at High. Meanwhile, tie turkey breast with a kitchen string horizontally, leaving approximately 2 inches apart. Season the meat with salt and pepper. Add the turkey to the pressure cooker and cook for about 3 minutes on each side. Transfer to a plate. Heat the remaining oil and cook shallots, thyme, garlic, and mushrooms until soft. Add white wine and scrape up the brown bits from the bottom. When the alcohol evaporates, return the turkey to the pressure cooker. Seal the lid, and cook on MEAT/STEW for 25 minutes at High.

Meanwhile, combine heavy cream and cornstarch in a small bowl. Do a quick pressure release. Open the lid and stir in the mixture. Bring the sauce to a boil, then turn the cooker off. Slice the turkey in half and serve topped with the creamy mushroom sauce.

Sweet Gingery and Garlicky Chicken Thighs

Ready in about: 25 minutes | Serves: 4 | Per serving: Calories 561; Carbs 61g; Fat 21g; Protein 54g

INGREDIENTS

2 pounds Chicken Thighs
½ cup Honey
3 tsp grated Ginger
2 tbsp Garlic, minced
5 tbsp Brown Sugar
2 cups Chicken Broth
½ cup plus 2 tbsp Soy Sauce
½ cup plus 2 tbsp Hoisin Sauce
4 tbsp Sriracha
2 tbsp Sesame Oil

DIRECTIONS

Lay the chicken at the bottom. Mix the remaining ingredients in a bowl. Pour the mixture over the chicken.

Seal the lid, select POULTRY and set the time to 20 minutes at High. Do a quick pressure release.

Simple Pressure Cooked Whole Chicken

Ready in about: 40 minutes | Serves: 4 | Per serving: Calories 376; Carbs 0g; Fat 30g; Protein 25g

INGREDIENTS

1 2-pound Whole Chicken
2 tbsp Olive Oil
1 ½ cups Water
Salt and Pepper, to taste

DIRECTIONS

Season chicken all over with salt and pepper. Heat the oil on SAUTÉ at High, and cook the chicken until browned on all sides. Set aside and wipe clean the cooker. Insert a rack in your pressure cooker and pour the water in. Lower the chicken onto the rack. Seal the lid. Choose POULTRY setting and adjust the time to 25 minutes at High pressure. Once the cooking is over, do a quick pressure release, by turning the valve to "open" position.

Chicken Bites Snacks with Chili Sauce

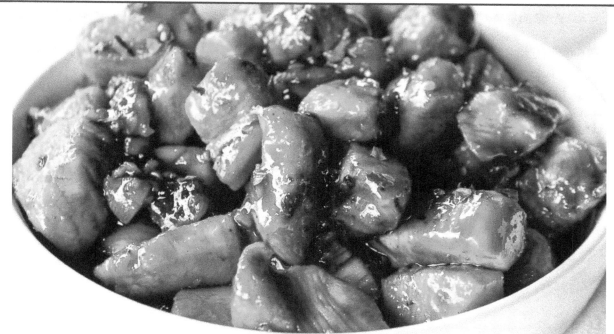

Ready in about: 25 minutes | Serves: 6 | Per serving: Calories 405; Carbs 18g; Fat 19g; Protein 31g

INGREDIENTS
1 ½ pounds Chicken, cut up, with bones
¼ cup Tomato Sauce
Kosher Salt and Black Pepper to taste
2 tsp dry Basil
¼ cup raw Honey
1 ½ cups Water
<u>FOR CHILI SAUCE:</u>
2 spicy Chili Peppers, halved
½ cup loosely packed Parsley, finely chopped
1 tsp Sugar
1 clove Garlic, chopped
2 tbsp Lime juice
¼ cup Olive Oil

DIRECTIONS
Put a steamer basket in the cooker's pot and pour the water in. Place the meat in the basket, and press BEANS/CHILI button. Seal the lid and cook for 20 minutes at High Pressure.

Meanwhile, prepare the sauce by mixing all the sauce ingredients in a food processor. Blend until the pepper is chopped and all the ingredients are mixed well. Release the pressure quickly. To serve, place the meat in serving bowl and top with the sauce.

Hot and Buttery Chicken Wings

Ready in about: 20 minutes | Serves: 16 | Per serving: Calories 50; Carbs 1g; Fat 2g; Protein 7g

INGREDIENTS

16 Chicken Wings
1 cup Hot Sauce
1 cup Water
2 tbsp Butter

DIRECTIONS

Add in all ingredients, and seal the lid. Cook on MEAT/STEW for 15 minutes at High. When ready, press CANCEL and release the pressure naturally, for 10 minutes.

Tasty Turkey with Campanelle and Tomato Sauce

Ready in about: 20 minutes | Serves: 4 | Per serving: Calories 588; Carbs 71g; Fat 11g; Protein 60g

INGREDIENTS

3 cups Tomato Sauce
½ tsp Salt
½ tbsp Marjoram
1 tsp dried Thyme
½ tbsp fresh Basil, chopped
¼ tsp ground Black Pepper, or more to taste
1 ½ pounds Turkey Breasts, chopped
1 tsp Garlic, minced
1 ½ cup spring Onions, chopped
1 package dry Campanelle Pasta
2 tbsp Olive Oil
½ cup Grana Padano cheese, grated

DIRECTIONS

Select SAUTÉ at High and heat the oil in the cooker. Place the turkey, spring onions and garlic. Cook until cooked, about 6-7 minutes. Add the remaining ingredients, except the cheese.

Seal the lid and press BEANS/CHILI button. Cook for 5 minutes at High Pressure. Once cooking has completed, quick release the pressure. To serve, top with freshly grated Grana Padano cheese.

Chicken with Mushrooms and Leeks

Ready in about: 25 minutes | Serves: 6 | Per serving: Calories 321; Carbs 31g; Fat 18g; Protein 39g

INGREDIENTS

2 pounds Chicken Breasts, cubed
4 tbsp Butter
1 ¼ pounds Mushrooms, sliced
½ cup Chicken Broth
2 tbsp Cornstarch
½ cup Milk
¼ tsp Black Pepper
2 Leeks, sliced
¼ tsp Garlic Powder

DIRECTIONS

Melt butter on SAUTÉ mode at High. Place chicken cubes inside and cook until they are no longer pink, and become slightly golden. Transfer the chicken pieces to a plate.

Add the leeks and sliced mushrooms to the pot and cook for about 3 minutes. Return the chicken to the pressure cooker, season with pepper and garlic powder, and pour in broth.

Give the mixture a good stir to combine everything well, then seal the lid. Set on BEANS/CHILI mode, for 8 minutes at High pressure. When it goes off, release the pressure quickly.

In a bowl, whisk together the milk and cornstarch. Pour the mixture over the chicken and set the pressure cooker to SAUTÉ at High. Cook until the sauce thickens.

Hearty and Hot Turkey Soup

Ready in about: 40 minutes | Serves: 6 | Per serving: Calories 398; Carbs 40g; Fat 11g; Protein 51g

INGREDIENTS

1 ½ pounds Turkey thighs, boneless, skinless and diced
1 cup Carrots, trimmed and diced
2 (8 oz) cans White Beans
2 Tomatoes, chopped
1 potato, chopped
1 cup Green Onions, chopped
2 Cloves Garlic, minced
6 cups Vegetable Stock
¼ tsp ground Black Pepper
¼ tsp Salt
½ tsp Cayenne Pepper
½ cup Celery head, peeled and chopped

DIRECTIONS

Place all ingredients, except the beans, into the pressure cooker, and select SOUP mode. Seal the lid and cook for 20 minutes at High Pressure. Release the pressure quickly.

Remove the lid and stir in the beans. Cover the cooker and let it stand for 10 minutes before serving.

Green BBQ Chicken Wings

Ready in about: 20 minutes | Serves: 4 | Per serving: Calories 311; Carbs 1g; Fat 10g; Protein 51g

INGREDIENTS

2 pounds Chicken Wings
5 tbsp Butter
1 cup Barbeque Sauce
5 Green Onions, minced

DIRECTIONS

Add the butter, ¾ parts of the sauce and chicken in the pressure cooker. Select POULTRY, seal the lid and cook for 15 minutes at High.

Do a quick release. Garnish wings with onions and top with the remaining sauce.

Hot and Spicy Shredded Chicken

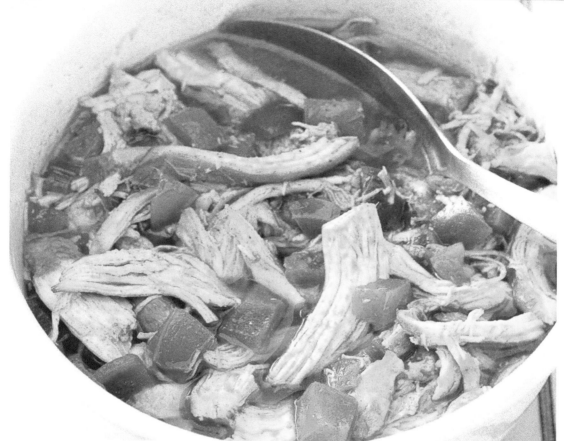

Ready in about: 1 hour | Serves: 4 | Per serving: Calories 307; Carbs 12g; Fat 10g; Protein 38g

INGREDIENTS

1 ½ pounds boneless and skinless Chicken Breasts
2 cups diced Tomatoes
½ tsp Oregano
2 Green Chilies, seeded and chopped
½ tsp Paprika
2 tbsp Coconut Sugar
½ cup Salsa
1 tsp Cumin
2 tbsp Olive Oil

DIRECTIONS

In a small mixing dish, combine the oil with all spices. Rub the chicken breast with the spicy marinade. Lay the meat into your pressure cooker. Add the tomatoes. Seal the lid, and cook for 20 minutes on POULTRY at High. Once ready, do a quick pressure release. Remove chicken to a cutting board; shred it. Return the shredded chicken to the cooker. Set to SAUTÉ at High, and let simmer for about 15 minutes.

Homemade Cajun Chicken Jambalaya

Ready in about: 30 minutes | Serves: 6 | Per serving: Calories 299; Carbs 31g; Fat 8g; Protein 41g

INGREDIENTS

1 ½ pounds, Chicken Breast, skinless
3 cups Chicken Stock
1 tbsp Garlic, minced
1 tsp Cajun Seasoning
1 Celery stalk, diced
1 ½ cups chopped Leeks, white part
1 ½ cups dry White Rice
2 tbsp Tomato Paste

DIRECTIONS

Select SAUTÉ at High and brown the chicken for 5 minutes. Add the garlic and celery, and fry for 2 minutes until fragrant. Deglaze with broth. Add the remaining ingredients to the cooker. Seal the lid.

Select POULTRY, and cook for 15 minutes at High. Do a quick pressure release and serve

Salsa and Lime Chicken with Rice

Ready in about: 35 minutes | Serves: 4 | Per serving: Calories 403; Carbs 44g; Fat 16g; Protein 19g

INGREDIENTS

¼ cup Lime Juice

3 tbsp Olive Oil

½ cup Salsa

2 Frozen Chicken Breasts, boneless and skinless

½ tsp Garlic Powder

1 cup Rice

1 cup Water

½ tsp Pepper

½ cup Mexican Cheese Blend

½ cup Tomato Sauce

DIRECTIONS

Lay the chicken into the pressure cooker. Pour lime juice, salt, garlic powder, olive oil, tomato sauce, and pepper, over the chicken. Seal the lid, and cook for 15 minutes on MEAT/STEW mode at High.

When ready, do a quick pressure release. Remove the chicken to a plate. Add in rice, cooking juices and water the total liquid in the pressure cooker should be about 2 cups.

Seal the lid and adjust the time to 10 minutes on BEANS/CHILI at High pressure. Do a quick pressure release and serve with cooked rice.

Homemade Whole Chicken

Ready in about: 40 minutes | Serves: 6 | Per serving: Calories 207; Carbs 1g; Fat 8g; Protein 29g

INGREDIENTS

3 - pound Whole Chicken
1 cup Chicken Broth
1 ½ tbsp Olive Oil
1 tsp Paprika
¾ tsp Garlic Powder
¼ tsp Onion Powder

DIRECTIONS

Rinse chicken under cold water, remove the giblets, and pat it dry with some paper towels. In a small bowl, combine the oil and spices. Rub the chicken well with the mixture. Set your pressure cooker to SAUTÉ at High. Add the chicken and sear on all sides until golden.

Pour the chicken broth around the chicken not over it), and seal the lid. Cook on BEANS/CHILI, for 25 minutes at High. Do a quick pressure release. Transfer the chicken to a platter and let sit for 10 minutes before carving.

Herbed and Garlicky Chicken Wings

Ready in about: 25 minutes | Serves: 4 | Per serving: Calories 177; Carbs 1g; Fat 10g; Protein 19g

INGREDIENTS
12 Chicken Wings
½ cup Chicken Broth
1 tbsp Basil
1 tbsp Oregano
½ tbsp Tarragon
1 tbsp Garlic, minced
2 tbsp Olive Oil
¼ tsp Pepper
1 cup Water

DIRECTIONS
Pour the water in the pressure cooker and lower the rack. Place all ingredients in a bowl and mix with your hands to combine well. Cover the bowl and let the wings sit for 15 minutes.

Arrange on the rack and seal the lid. Select BEANS/CHILI, and set the timer to 10 minutes at High pressure. When done, do a quick pressure release. Serve drizzled with the cooking liquid and enjoy!

Duck and Green Pea Soup

Ready in about: 30 minutes | Serves: 6 | Per serving: Calories 191; Carbs 14g; Fat 5g; Protein 21g

INGREDIENTS

1 cup Carrots, diced
4 cups Chicken Stock
1 pound Duck Breasts, chopped
20 ounces diced canned Tomatoes
1 cup Celery, chopped
18 ounces Green Peas
1 cup Onions, diced
2 Garlic Cloves, minced
1 tsp dried Marjoram
½ tsp Pepper
½ tsp Salt

DIRECTIONS

Place all ingredients, except the peas, in your pressure cooker. Stir well to combine and seal the lid. Select SOUP mode and set the cooking time to 20 minutes at High.

After the beep, do a quick pressure release. Stir in the peas. Seal the lid again but do NOT turn the pressure cooker on. Let blanch for about 7 minutes. Ladle into serving bowls.

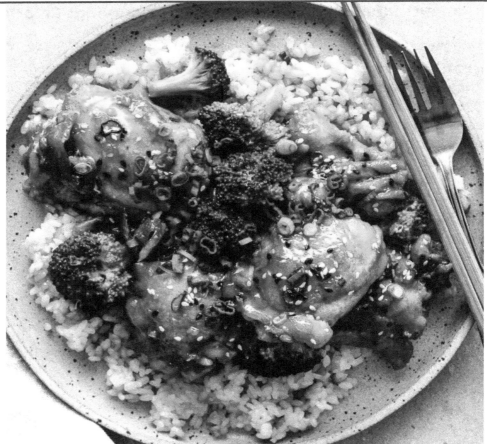

Ready in about: 25 minutes | Serves: 8 | Per serving: Calories 352; Carbs 31g; Fat 11g; Protein 31g

INGREDIENTS

1 cup Chicken Broth
¾ cup Brown Sugar
2 tbsp ground Ginger
1 tsp Pepper
3 pounds Boneless and Skinless Chicken Thighs
¼ cup Apple Cider Vinegar
¾ cup low-sodium Soy Sauce
20 ounces canned Pineapple, crushed
2 tbsp Garlic Powder

DIRECTIONS

Stir all of the ingredients, except for the chicken. Add the chicken meat and turn to coat. Seal the lid, press POULTRY and cook for 20 minutes at High. Do a quick pressure release, by turning the valve to "open" position.

Young Goose for Slow Cooker

The mild taste of wild goose!

Prep time: 21 minutes Cooking time: 6 hours Servings: 6

INGREDIENTS:

3 tbsp fresh rosemary
Chopped celery
Cream of mushroom soup
Fresh sage
2 goose
Cream of celery soup
Fresh thyme
Cream of chicken soup
1 cup mushrooms
1 pack baby carrots

DIRECTIONS:

Finely mince fresh thyme, rosemary, and sage leaves. Chop celery and baby carrots.

In a wide bowl, mix cream of celery, carrots, cream of chicken soup. Celery, cream of mushroom soup, sage, thyme, mushrooms and rosemary.

Cut goose into pieces and place into Slow Cooker. Pour the cream mixture over the meat.

Set to HIGH and cook for 8 hours until tender.

Nutrition: Calories: 998 Fat: 56g Carbohydrates: 17g Protein: 91g

Homemade Chicken with Dumplings

Try this freshly cooked chicken with your family!

Prep time: 21 minutes Cooking time: 6 hours Servings: 6

INGREDIENTS:

1 cup water

4 cans chicken broth

4 carrots

Salt

2 tbsp flour

4 baking potatoes

2 cups baking mix

2 cups chopped broccoli

Black pepper

4 tbsp milk

DIRECTIONS:

Right in Slow Cooker, mix potatoes, chicken meat, broccoli and carrots.

In a separate bowl, mix water and flour until it appears to be paste-like.

Season with pepper and salt to taste.

Pour in over the Slow Cooker ingredients and stir well. Cover and cook for 5 hours on LOW mode.

In small bowl, combine baking mix and milk. Carefully add to Slow Cooker, using a teaspoon. Cook for another hour.

Nutrition: Calories: 649 Fat: 22g Carbohydrates: 62g Protein: 47g

Mexican-styled Slow Cooker Chicken

Add this to your tacos and salads, or just serve with pasta or rice!

Prep time: 11 minutes Cooking time: 4 hours Servings: 4

INGREDIENTS:

Half cup tomato salsa

Half cup tomato preserves

Half cup chipotle salsa

One chicken

DIRECTIONS:

In a bowl, mix pineapple preserves, chipotle salsa and tomato salsa. If needed, remove skin and bones from the chicken meat.

Place chicken into Slow Cooker and pour over with the sauce. Toss meat to cover evenly. Cook for 3 hours on LOW mode.

Remove chicken meat from Slow Cooker and finely shred with two forks. Return to Slow Cooker and prepare for 1 more hour.

Nutrition: Calories: 238 Fat: 2g Carbohydrates: 31g Protein: 23g

Yellow Rice with Turkey wings

Quick and easy for working days!

Prep time: 21 minutes Cooking time: 6 hours Servings: 6

INGREDIENTS:

1 tsp seasoned salt
3 turkey wings
1 tsp garlic powder
Ground black pepper
Water to cover
Cream of mushroom soup
1 pack saffron rice

DIRECTIONS:

Clean the turkey wings and transfer to Slow Cooker.

In a bowl, mix garlic powder, salt, cream of mushroom soup, black pepper. Season the wings with this mixture.

Pour in water into Slow Cooker – just enough to cover the wings. Stir everything well and cover. Cook for 8 hours on LOW mode.

When it is time, stir the rice into Slow Cooker and prepare for 20 minutes more.

Nutrition: Calories: 272 Fat: 5g Carbohydrates: 39g Protein: 17g

Slow Cooker Turkey Wings

You can try it with your favorite sauce and side dishes!

Prep time: 11 minutes Cooking time: 7 hours Servings: 12

INGREDIENTS:

Salt

Ground black pepper

6 turkey legs

3 tsp poultry seasoning

DIRECTIONS:

Wash the turkey legs with running water and remove excess liquid.

Rub each turkey leg with one teaspoon of poultry seasoning. Add salt and black pepper. Cut aluminum foil into leg-fitting parts and wrap each turkey leg with a foil.

Place the wrapped legs into Slow Cooker. Add no water or other liquids.

Cook on LOW for 8 hours. Check the tenderness before serving.

Nutrition: Calories: 217 Fat: 7g Carbohydrates: 1g Protein: 36g

Chicken Alfredo in Slow Cooker

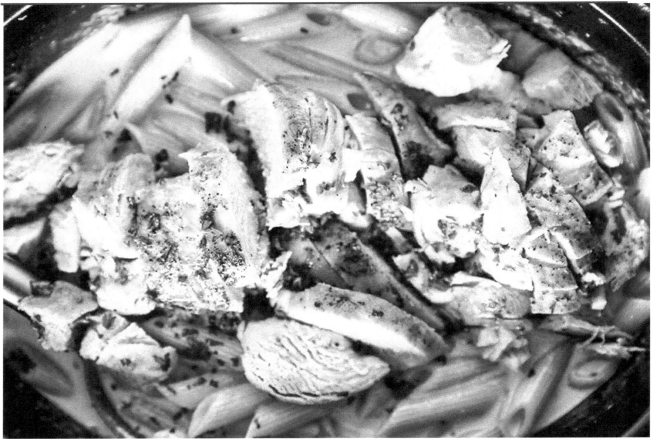

Easy with Alfredo sauce and Swiss cheese!

Prep time: 16 minutes Cooking time: 4 hours Servings: 6

INGREDIENTS:

Black pepper
3 tbsp grated Parmesan cheese
4 chicken breast halves
Salt
4 slices Swiss cheese
Garlic powder

DIRECTIONS:

Wash your chicken breasts with running water. Remove the bones and skin. Cut chicken meat into small cubes.

Right in Slow Cooker, combine chicken cubes and Alfredo sauce. Toss to cover. Cook under lid on LOW mode, approximately for two hours.

Add both cheeses and cook for another 30 minutes.

Just before serving, season with salt, garlic powder and black pepper to taste.

Nutrition: Calories: 610 Fat: 50g Carbohydrates: 9g Protein: 31g

It will wait for you to come home!

Prep time: 16 minutes Cooking time: 8 hours Servings: 6

INGREDIENTS:

Half cup sour cream

4 chicken breast halves

Cream of celery

Cream of chicken soup

DIRECTIONS:

Discard the skin and bones from the chicken. Wash and drain.

Grease your Slow Cooker with melted butter or olive oil. If you prefer cooking spray, use it. Transfer cleared chicken into Slow Cooker.

In a bowl, whisk both creams. Mix well until smooth. Pour the chicken meat with cream mixture.

Cover with the lid and prepare for 8 hours on LOW mode. Just before serving, add the sour cream.

To serve, transfer cooked chicken onto a large bowl. Garnish with chopped green onion or other vegetables or berries. Serve hot.

Nutrition: Calories: 304 Fat: 16g Carbohydrates: 12g Protein: 27g

Slow Cooker Turkey with Dumplings

Creamy and hot, perfect choice for a cold day!

Prep time: 9 minutes Cooking time: 4 hours Servings: 4

INGREDIENTS:

3 medium carrots
1 cans cream of chicken soup
Garlic powder
1 can chicken broth
Half onion
Buttermilk biscuit dough
5 large potatoes
2 tbsp butter
Cooked turkey
Poultry seasoning

DIRECTIONS:

Cook the turkey before start.

Chop the potatoes, onion and carrots.

In a bowl, mix butter, onion, potatoes, turkey, chicken broth and cream of chicken soup. Season with garlic powder.

Transfer into Slow Cooker and pour in water to cover. Cook on HIGH mode for 3 hours, stirring occasionally. Place the biscuits over turkey and cook for 1 more hour

Nutrition: Calories: 449 Fat: 22g Carbohydrates: 38g Protein: 23g

Flavored Chicken in Rustic Italian Style

Perfect with veggies and Italian seasoning!

Prep time: 22 minutes Cooking time: 5 hours Servings: 6

INGREDIENTS:

3 cups penne pasta
Red bell pepper
Chicken thighs
Canned tomatoes
Salt
Canned crushed tomatoes
Black pepper
Fresh mushrooms
2 carrots
4 garlic cloves

DIRECTIONS:

Grease Slow Cooker with oil or spray with anti-stick cooking spray. Transfer chicken to Slow Cooker.

Chop carrots into 1-inch slices, slice bell peppers and mushrooms. Mice garlic.

Add the vegetables and add canned tomatoes, salt/pepper and season with two tablespoons of Italian seasoning.

Cover and cook on LOW for 8 hours.

To serve, use 3 cups penne pasta or fresh parsley.

Nutrition: Calories: 441 Fat: 16g Carbohydrates: 41g Protein: 31g

Hot Turkey Meatballs

Perfectly to serve with vegetables!

Prep time: 17 minutes Cooking time: 3 hours Servings: 4

INGREDIENTS:

Water
Dry onion soup mix (2 envelopes)
2 Chicken eggs
Beef flavored rice
Fresh turkey meat

DIRECTIONS:

Fill your Slow Cooker with water and onion soup mix (there should be enough liquid to fill crockpot halfway).

Turn on Slow Cooker to high and leave until the liquid boils.

Meanwhile, make meatballs. In a bowl, combine rice with turkey and flavoring mix. Add beaten chicken eggs and mix together.

Form 2-inch meatballs and fry them to brown on large skillet with oil.

When soup is boiling. Transfer meatballs to Slow Cooker and prepare 9 hours on LOW temperature mode.

Nutrition: Calories: 567 Fat: 22g Carbohydrates: 42g Protein: 47g

Shredded Turkey in Barbeque Sauce

Full of protein and healthy meal!

Prep time: 13 minutes Cooking time: 10 hours Servings: 8

INGREDIENTS:

1 tsp ground cumin
8 potato rolls
2 cans baked beans
1 medium onion
1 tbsp yellow mustard
2 bone-in turkey thighs
salt

DIRECTIONS:

Finely chop onion.
Grease your Slow Cooker with melted plain butter.
Right in Slow Cooker pot, combine onion, baked beans, barbeque sauce, cumin, yellow mustard and salt.
Carefully place the turkey thighs into the mixture.
Set Slow Cooker to LOW temperature and cook for 11 hours.
Remove turkey and discard bones. Shred and place back to Slow Cooker.
Serve the turkey placed over potato rolls.

Nutrition: Calories: 385 Fat: 6g Carbohydrates: 59g Protein: 26g

Lemon-Fragrant Chicken

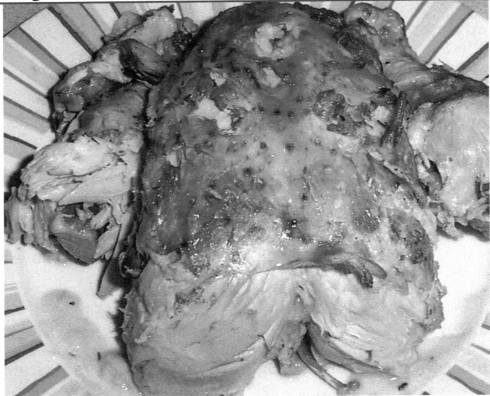

Easy and great to taste!

Prep time: 22 minutes Cooking time: 9 hours Servings: 6

INGREDIENTS:
1 medium onion
1 cup hot water
Salt
One stalk celery
One whole chicken
One big apple
Half tsp dried rosemary
zest and juice of 1 lemon
ground black pepper

DIRECTIONS:
Peel and core apple. Cut into quarters.
Wash the chicken and dry with a paper towel.
Rub the salt and pepper mix into chickens' skin and place apple and chopped celery into chicken. Place chicken into Slow Cooker and sprinkle with chopped onion, lemon zest and juice, rosemary. Pour in one cup water.
Cover and cook on HIGH for 1 hour. Then, turn to LOW and cook for 7 hours.

Nutrition: Calories: 309 Fat: 17g Carbohydrates: 7g Protein: 31g

Turkey with Indian Spice

Perfect with rice and fresh herbs!

Prep time: 17 minutes Cooking time: 6 hours Servings: 4

INGREDIENTS:

Turkey thigh meat
Canned stewed tomatoes
3 tbsp dried onion flakes
Dried thyme leaves
4 tbsp white wine
Half tsp Italian seasoning
6 cubes chicken bouillon
Garlic powder
Lemon pepper seasoning

DIRECTIONS:

In a bowl, whisk together wine and canned tomatoes.

Pour in the tomato mixture into your Slow Cooker and add onion flakes, bouillon cubes and thyme. Season with garlic powder and Italian seasoning.

Carefully place the turkey into Slow Cooker.

Cover the lid and cook for 10 hours on LOW temperature mode.

Nutrition: Calories: 317 Fat: 7g Carbohydrates: 9g Protein: 51g

Gluten-free Chicken Soup

Easy to cook on a busy day!

Prep time: 13 minutes Cooking time: 8 hours Servings: 9

INGREDIENTS:

Medium onion

1/2 cup water

2 carrots

Gluten-free chicken broth

Salt

Frozen vegetables

4 tbsp. long-grain rice

2 celery stalks

Garlic

Black pepper

Dried basil

tomatoes

Red pepper flakes

DIRECTIONS:

In a bowl, combine diced tomatoes, diced carrots, garlic, celery and onions. Transfer the vegetable mix into Slow Cooker and season with dried basil, red pepper flakes, salt and pepper.

Carefully place chicken into the mixture. Stir everything well to cover the meat. Cook on LOW temperature mode for 7 hours.

Add rice and frozen vegetable mix. Cook for 1 more hour on HIGH.

Nutrition: Calories: 198 Fat: 6g Carbohydrates: 20g Protein: 16g

Hawaiian Spice Slow Cooker Chicken

Amazingly tastes with rice!

Prep time: 5 minutes Cooking time: 4 hours Servings: 9

INGREDIENTS:

Chicken breasts
Canned sliced pineapples
1 tsp soy sauce
1 bottle honey bbq sauce

DIRECTIONS:

Carefully grease the bottom and sides of your Slow Cooker with melted butter or spray with anti- stick spray.

Wash and drain chicken breasts, place into Slow Cooker.

In a bowl, mix pineapple slices and barbeque sauce, add soy sauce. Pour in this mixture over chicken breasts into Slow Cooker.

Cover the lid and turn Slow Cooker to HIGH temperature mode. Cook for 5 hours. To serve, garnish chicken with chopped parsley and green onion. Serve while hot.

Nutrition: Calories: 274 Fat: 3g Carbohydrates: 29g Protein: 30g

Chicken Soup with Rice

Your whole family will like this soup!

Prep time: 5 minutes Cooking time: 8 hours Servings: 6

INGREDIENTS:

3 celery sticks
4 tbsp long-grain rice
2 cups frozen mixed vegetables
Half cup water
1 tbsp dried parsley
Lemon seasoning
3 cans chicken broth
Herb seasoning

DIRECTIONS:

Remove bones from chicken breast halves. Cook and dice the meat. In a bowl, combine chopped celery, rice, mixed vegetables.

Season the mixture with lemon and herbal seasoning. Add some salt to taste and transfer to Slow Cooker.

Whisk water and chicken broth; pour over the vegetable and chicken mixture in Slow Cooker. Cover and cook for 8 hours, using LOW temperature mode.

Nutrition: Calories: 277 Fat: 7g Carbohydrates: 27g Protein: 25g

Tunisian-Styled Turkey

Satisfying and tasty dish for any holiday!

Prep time: 11 minutes Cooking time: 4 hours Servings: 6

INGREDIENTS:

2 tbsp flour
1 turkey breast half
Chipotle chili powder
1 tbsp olive oil
Half tsp garlic powder
1 acorn squash
Ground cinnamon
3 large carrots
Coriander
2 red onions
Salt
6 garlic cloves
Ground black pepper

DIRECTIONS:

Mix chipotle and garlic powder, black pepper, cinnamon and salt.

Rub turkey meat with spicy mix and brown in a large skillet (use medium heat). Grease your Slow Cooker with olive oil.

Cover the bottom of Slow Cooker with diced carrots, acorn squash quarters, garlic cloves and red onions.

Place the turkey atop the vegetables. Cook on HIGH mode for 8 hours.

Nutrition: Calories: 455 Fat: 5g Carbohydrates: 19g Protein: 81g

Hot Buffalo Chicken Lettuce Envelopes

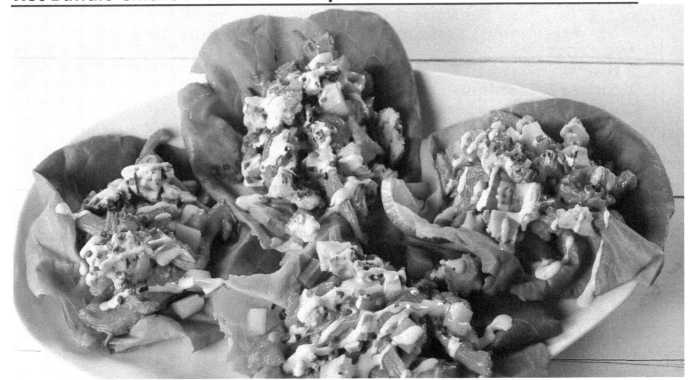

So much healthier than traditional Buffalo wings!

Prep time: 11 minutes Cooking time: 6 hours Servings: 10

INGREDIENTS:

2 chicken breasts
1 pack ranch dressing mix
One head Boston lettuce leaves
Cayenne pepper sauce

DIRECTIONS:

Remove skin and bones from the chicken and put the breasts into Slow Cooker.

In a bowl, stir to smooth ranch dressing mix and cayenne pepper. Stir the mixture until it is smooth.

Pour the chicken breasts with the sauce. Make sure that all the chicken surface is covered with the sayce.

Cover and cook during 7 hours (use LOW temperature mode).

Using spotted spoon, place chicken meat over the lettuce leaves and roll.

Nutrition: Calories: 105 Fat: 2g Carbohydrates: 2g Protein: 18g

Chicken with Pear and Asparagus

Unusual seasoning for incredibly tasty dish!

Prep time: 21 minutes Cooking time: 4 hours Servings: 4

INGREDIENTS:

4 cloves garlic
1 tbsp vegetable oil
2 tbsp balsamic vinegar
4 chicken breast halves
3 tbsp apple juice
One onion
Dried rosemary
Black pepper, salt
Grated fresh ginger
Two Bartlett pears
2 tbsp brown sugar
Fresh asparagus

DIRECTIONS:

Core and slice Bartlett pears.

Warm the olive on preheated skillet. Cook chicken meat until it is completely browned. Transfer to Slow Cooker.

Dice the onion and spread it over the chicken. Season with salt and pepper. Place asparagus and pears into Slow Cooker.

Separately mix balsamic vinegar, sugar, apple juice, sugar, ginger and garlic. Add to Slow Cooker. Cover and cook for 5 hours on LOW mode.

Nutrition: Calories: 309 Fat: 7g Carbohydrates: 33g Protein: 29g

Sweet Chicken with Parmesan

This one will be your favorite!

Prep time: 11 minutes Cooking time: 5 hours Servings: 6

INGREDIENTS:

Black pepper
6 tbsp butter
Salt to taste
Onion soup mix
Cream of mushroom soup
Grated Parmesan
1 cup milk
1 cup rice
6 chicken breasts

DIRECTIONS:

Remove skin and bones off the chicken.

Separately mix milk, onion soup mix, rice and cream of mushroom soup.

Slightly grease Slow Cooker, lay chicken meat over the bottom.

Pour the sauce mixture all over it.

In addition, season with pepper/salt.

Finally, cover with grated Parmesan cheese.

Set Slow Cooker to LOW and prepare for 10 hours.

Nutrition: Calories: 493 Fat: 21g Carbohydrates: 37g Protein: 35g

Cornish Hens with Olives

Perfect with wild rice or vegetables!

Prep time: 21 minutes Cooking time: 4 hours Servings: 2

INGREDIENTS:

1 tsp garlic salt
2 Cornish game hens
One large zucchini
Golden mushroom soup
Pimento-stuffed green olives
Baby Portobello mushrooms

DIRECTIONS:

To start, prepare the vegetables: chop zucchini, mushrooms and green olives. Slightly coat the hens with 3 tablespoons of golden mushroom soup. In a bowl, mix olives, remaining mushroom soup, garlic salt and zucchini. Stuff the hens with this mixture.

Transfer hens into Slow Cooker and pour over with some more mushroom soup (all that remained).

Set your Slow Cooker to HIGH mode and cook for 4 hours.

Nutrition: Calories: 851 Fat: 57g Carbohydrates: 24g Protein: 59g

Chicken Livers Mix

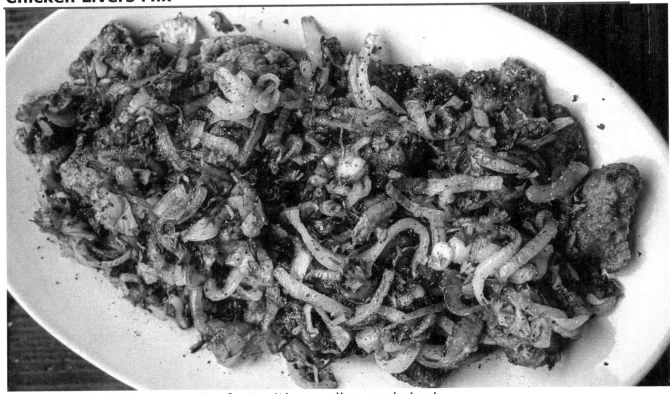

Perfect with noodles and rice!

Prep time: 34 minutes Cooking time: 6-7 hours Servings: 4

INGREDIENTS:
3 green onions
1 tsp salt
Dry white wine
3 slices bacon
Black pepper
One cup chicken stock
Canned sliced mushrooms
1 pound chicken livers
Golden mushroom soup

DIRECTIONS:
In a medium bowl, mix salt, flour and pepper. Place livers into this mixture and toss to cover. Cook bacon on a skillet, over the medium heat). Remove and drain with paper towels.

Place the livers into the same skillet and cook until lightly browned. Place the livers and bacon into Slow Cooker. Pour in the chicken stock. Add golden mushroom soup and wine.

Cook under the lid for 6 hours. Use LOW temperature mode.

Nutrition: Calories: 352 Fat: 16g Carbohydrates: 21g Protein: 24g

we have actually come to the end of this fantastic and also rich Crock Pot pressure cooker.

Did you take pleasure in trying these brand-new and tasty recipes?

we truly wish so, and also a lot more will certainly show up soon.

To highlight the renovations, constantly integrated with our tasty and also healthy and balanced recipes of exercise, this is a guidance that we intend to give due to the fact that we consider it the most effective mix. a huge hug as well as we will certainly be back soon to maintain you company with our recipes. See you quickly.

CPSIA information can be obtained
at www.ICGtesting.com
Printed in the USA
LVHW062315230521
688301LV00006B/346